Praise for *The Doctor's Guide to Gastrointestinal Health*

"This is the reference guide you dream about—answers to all your important questions, written in a language you can understand. For everyone who wants better health and peace of mind."

—Diane Sawyer, co-anchor of ABCNews' *Good Morning America* and *Primetime Thursday*

"An important, practical, easy-to-read and understand source of information for anyone with a chronic gastrointestinal problem."

—Isadore Rosenfeld, M.D., attending physician at New York–Presbyterian Hospital and Memorial Sloan Kettering Cancer Center, Rossi Distinguished Professor of Clinical Medicine at Weill Cornell Medical Center, and bestselling author

"This book will provide for patients and their relatives authoritative, up-to-date information about most diseases of the gastrointestinal tract. The disorders are clearly explained and available treatments are outlined in clear language. Of special importance is the description of various diagnostic procedures used in gastroenterology, together with important information about what patients can expect before, during and after these treatments. This should go a long way toward relieving the anxiety that accompanies diagnostic procedures."

—Jeremiah A. Barondess, M.D., president of The New York Academy of Medicine

"As a long time patient of Dr. Miskovitz, I highly recommend *The Doctor's Guide to Gastrointestinal Health* for anyone wanting to know the vital importance of preventative procedures—before it's too late. My wife and I have gone to Dr. Miskovitz for all our procedures and we're still here—thanks in part to an early diagnosis."

—Warner Wolf, TV and radio sportscaster and author of *Let's Go to the Videotape: All the Plays and Replays from My Life in Sports*

The Doctor's Guide to Gastrointestinal Health

The Doctor's Guide to Gastrointestinal Health

Preventing and Treating Acid Reflux, Ulcers,
Irritable Bowel Syndrome, Diverticulitis,
Celiac Disease, Colon Cancer, Pancreatitis,
Cirrhosis, Hernias, and More

Paul Miskovitz, M.D.
Weill Medical College of Cornell University,
New York–Presbyterian Hospital

Marian Betancourt

WILEY

John Wiley & Sons, Inc.

For our families

Copyright © 2005 by Paul Miskovitz, M.D., and Marian Betancourt. All rights reserved

Published by John Wiley & Sons, Inc., Hoboken, New Jersey
Published simultaneously in Canada

Design and composition by Navta Associates, Inc.

No part of this publication may be reproduced, stored in a retrieval system, or transmitted in any form or by any means, electronic, mechanical, photocopying, recording, scanning, or otherwise, except as permitted under Section 107 or 108 of the 1976 United States Copyright Act, without either the prior written permission of the Publisher, or authorization through payment of the appropriate per-copy fee to the Copyright Clearance Center, 222 Rosewood Drive, Danvers, MA 01923, (978) 750-8400, fax (978) 646-8600, or on the web at www.copyright.com. Requests to the Publisher for permission should be addressed to the Permissions Department, John Wiley & Sons, Inc., 111 River Street, Hoboken, NJ 07030, (201) 748-6011, fax (201) 748-6008.

Limit of Liability/Disclaimer of Warranty: While the publisher and the author have used their best efforts in preparing this book, they make no representations or warranties with respect to the accuracy or completeness of the contents of this book and specifically disclaim any implied warranties of merchantability or fitness for a particular purpose. No warranty may be created or extended by sales representatives or written sales materials. The advice and strategies contained herein may not be suitable for your situation. You should consult with a professional where appropriate. Neither the publisher nor the author shall be liable for any loss of profit or any other commercial damages, including but not limited to special, incidental, consequential, or other damages.

The information contained in this book is not intended to serve as a replacement for professional medical advice. Any use of the information in this book is at the reader's discretion. The author and publisher specifically disclaim any and all liability arising directly or indirectly from the use or application of any information contained in this book. A health-care professional should be consulted regarding your specific situation.

For general information about our other products and services, please contact our Customer Care Department within the United States at (800) 762-2974, outside the United States at (317) 572-3993 or fax (317) 572-4002.

Wiley also publishes its books in a variety of electronic formats. Some content that appears in print may not be available in electronic books. For more information about Wiley products, visit our web site at www.wiley.com.

Library of Congress Cataloging-in-Publication Data:

Miskovitz, Paul F., date
  The doctor's guide to gastrointestinal health : preventing and treating acid reflux, ulcers, irritable bowel syndrome, diverticulitis, celiac disease, colon cancer, pancreatitis, cirrhosis, hernias, and more / Paul Miskovitz, Marian Betancourt.
    p. cm.
  Includes bibliographical references and index.
  ISBN 0-471-46237-3 (pbk.)
  1. Gastrointestinal system—Diseases—Popular works. I. Betancourt, Marian. II. Title.
RC806.M57 2005
616.3'3—dc22   2004027081

Printed in the United States of America

10 9 8 7 6 5 4 3 2 1

Contents

Introduction

In today's managed health-care system, doctors have less time to educate their patients. At the same time, these patients have access to reams of health information on the Internet, but much of it can be more harmful than no information at all. With this book we hope to fill an urgent need for an easy-to-use but comprehensive book that helps you understand how the gastrointestinal system works and how to take care of it.

Digestive ailments—whether mild or life-threatening—can be difficult to diagnose and treat. Thus the field is surrounded by a lot of quasi-medical information and treatment, such as high colonic enemas, bio-ecological diets, and other fad diets that can cause real harm to your health. People sometimes resort to chiropractors, hypnotists, nutritionists, and self-medication instead of continuing their search for the correct medical diagnosis.

The Doctor's Guide to Gastrointestinal Health is meant to inform you about diagnostic and treatment options available, so you know what questions to ask your doctor before any treatment begins.

In Part I, there's an overview of how the gastrointestinal system works and how it is affected by lifestyle, age, and the mind. A section on common symptoms will help you know when you need medical attention. The role of the gastroenterologist and diagnostic testing is well covered, along with an entire chapter on endoscopic procedures that have transformed gastroenterology. There's also important information about medical insurance coverage of these procedures.

Part II details causes, symptoms, diagnoses, and medical treatments for all of the disorders and diseases of the gastrointestinal system. It covers everything from top to bottom, in that order: esophagus, stomach, small intestine, gallbladder, pancreas, liver, colon and rectum, and the abdominal cavity.

And finally, Part III is a commonsense guide to maintaining a healthy gastrointestinal system, with guidelines for diet and exercise, checkups and screenings, as well as some precautions to take when you travel to other parts of the world.

In making *The Doctor's Guide to Gastrointestinal Health* as comprehensive as possible, we hope it serves as a useful resource for you and your family. No matter what your concern or condition may be, this book will help you identify and treat the problem, and in many cases, help you prevent it.

PART I

Understanding How Your Gut Works and How to Identify Problems

Chapter 1

What We Know about the Gut:
Yesterday, Today, and Tomorrow

OUR EARLY ANCESTORS probably never had the digestive problems we have today, even though they ate anything and everything they could find. While animals are generally pretty picky about what they eat, early humans had a diverse diet of nuts, berries, plants, fish, animals, bugs—you name it. And they ate the nutrient-rich stems, pits, roots, and husks of this matter as well.

When we evolved from hunter-gathering to agriculture, we added grains to our diet. With industrialization, mills refined our grains, removing the husks, bran, and cereal germ—and most of the nutrients along with it. Civilization led us toward food in boxes and packages from the shelves of supermarkets. Few people knew or cared about what was in that box or the consequences of eating its contents.

Our awareness has improved somewhat. Most of us now realize how poor nutrition and lack of exercise have lead to the obesity epidemic and a plethora of chronic digestive diseases. The shift in diet, along with smoking, drinking, and stress in the past hundred years, are directly related to the problems we face today. The good news is that we have the tools to diagnose digestive diseases early and have the means to cure many that were not curable in the past, such as peptic ulcers, celiac disease, and lactose intolerance.

Gastroenterology has developed into an amazingly precise discipline with the impact of technology and the evolution of concepts of specific diseases. We now understand gut secretions and gut hormones. We know how dietary elements are transported. As early as 1881, Polish surgeon Jan Mikulicz-Radecki used the first prototype "scope" to look into the esophagus. The development of fiberoptic endoscopy by Dr. Basil Isaac Hirschowitz gave us the tools to look inside the digestive tract and take away tissue samples or remove polyps. We learned that bacteria, not stress, in many cases caused stomach ulcers. In the 1980s an Australian physician, Barry Marshall, was so convinced ulcers were caused by *H. pylori* bacterium that he swallowed bacteria to prove his point to skeptical colleagues. While still a resident physician seventy-five years ago, Robert Elman discovered a way to diagnose that someone had pancreatitis. Some of the early heroes, with no sophisticated tools but their own curiosity and imagination, gave us other breakthroughs.

How the Digestive System Works

The digestive system sends us messages all the time. Our stomachs growl when we are hungry. We feel a burning sensation in our esophagus or stomach when we eat something irritating. We feel a knot in our stomach when we are upset. We might have a gut reaction to some encounters in our lives. We get a very particular urge when we have to go to the bathroom. All of these signals come from a complex system of dynamics that involves our entire physiology—blood, nerves, hormones, muscles—and its interaction with the brain.

A series of involuntary, wavelike muscle contractions propels your food in one direction along the alimentary tract—from the mouth to the anus. This action is called peristalsis. When your stomach gurgles, it is the sound of these peristaltic contractions propelling food along, an action you cannot feel. In the stomach, peristalsis produces a churning action that aids digestion. Circular muscles called sphincters are at the entrance to the esophagus and at the exits from the esophagus, the stomach, the lower small intestine, and the rectum, or anal opening. These muscles close tightly to prevent the process from going in reverse and causing one to vomit.

On its trip through the alimentary tract, food is broken down. Starches become simple sugars. Fats change to fatty acids and glycerin. Proteins become amino acids. The salivary glands in the mouth produce lubrication and enzymes and begin this conversion. The stomach stores and digests about one quart of food. Stomach muscles churn and mix with gastric juice, which includes hydrochloric acid and pepsin.

Within two to five hours, the digested food passes from the stomach to the duodenum, the first section of the small intestine. The small intestine is a twenty-plus-foot-long narrow, muscular tube—like a coiled soft rubber hose—that is made up of layers called the mucosa, the submucosa, and the serosa. The main function of the small intestine is the further digestion and absorption of nutrients. Also, enzymes from the pancreas, alkaline juices, and bile emulsifiers made by the liver and stored in the gallbladder enter the system at the duodenum level. Bile acids help dissolve (solubilize) dietary fats the way detergent dissolves grease in dishwater.

Most absorption, as well as digestion, occurs in the small intestine. Nutrients are absorbed into lymph fluids or blood vessels in the intestine wall (across the mucosa). Whatever cannot be digested in the small intestine, such as plant fiber, empties into the cecum at the lower right side of the abdomen. The cecum is the beginning of the large intestine, or colon. The colon, only about five feet long, is shorter than the small intestine but it is much wider (the girth is responsible for the label large intestine). The colon, positioned like a question mark, partially encircles the small intestine.

The main function of the large intestine is to absorb salt and water from all the remaining digested food that has been passed from the small intestine. In a healthy adult, more than a gallon of water, with more than an ounce of salt, is absorbed from the colon every four hours. Bacteria in the colon then convert fecal matter into its final form.

Digested matter travels upward from the cecum into the ascending colon, across the abdomen in the transverse colon, down the left side of the abdomen in the descending and s-shaped sigmoid colon, and into the rectum, where the solid waste is stored until it is eliminated. In doing this job, the colon produces a variety of substances, including carbon dioxide, hydrogen, methane, and the billions of bacteria that live in the colon.

All of this coiled tubing is supported by the mesentery, a membrane-like fold of tissue attached to the back of the abdominal cavity. The mesentery contains blood vessels, nerves, and the lymph system that interacts with the intestines.

Digestion and the absorption of nutrients into the bloodstream are as effortless as breathing and normally produce no sensations such as pain. Most discomfort in the gastrointestinal tract occurs in the two main storage areas: the stomach and the colon. When you feel discomfort above the waist, it is often in your esophagus, stomach, or duodenum, all close to the heart. Thus indigestion is often called heartburn. Discomfort below the waist usually means a problem in the colon, such as constipation or diarrhea.

Your Second Brain: The Mind-Gut Connection

Nervous stomach, gut-wrenching, gut reaction—these are all common terms. We understand them on a gut level without really thinking about how these terms came to be. A case of nerves before making a speech could have you running to the bathroom. A shocking piece of news could make someone throw up. Because of this mysterious connection, people were sometimes told that their digestive problems were all in their mind when they could not be diagnosed or treated effectively. The interaction between body and mind was overemphasized in the past. For example, it was once believed that ulcers were caused by stress. Today we know that while bacteria cause most ulcers, some can be caused by nonsteroidal anti-inflammatory drugs or by gut hormone imbalances such as gastrinoma (Zollinger-Ellison Syndrome).

The gut is, in fact, the center of the enteric nervous system. Nerves travel from the brain to the esophagus, stomach, gallbladder, pancreas, small intestine, and colon. This is why the smell or sight of food can stimulate stomach and intestinal contractions. It also can stimulate stomach acid and pancreatic enzyme secretions.

In the same way, when you are stressed and your nerves are on maximum overload, the ones in your digestive system can cause cramps, too much acid secretion, and other problems. Some of us can handle stress with nary a twitch in our enteric nervous system, but others cannot. Some are so sensitive that they become predisposed to conditions that work hand in hand with such stress, such as irritable bowel syndrome (see chapter 10). In 2000 Michael D. Gershon explained much of this fascinating system—neurogastroenterology—in *The Second Brain: A Groundbreaking New Understanding of Nervous Disorders of the Stomach and Intestine*.

There is a reason for every disorder, whether or not we can find an organic cause. In fact, digestive disorders are always classified as organic or functional. Organic means it comes from a disease state such as a faulty valve between the esophagus and the stomach, which diagnostic tests can find. When something isn't working properly but we can't find any structural or organic damage, then it is called a functional disorder. This could be subtle defects in the chemistry of the system, or that the system is not coordinating. These distinctions make diagnosis and treatment more challenging. Organic problems such as an inflamed colon can be treated with medication and change in diet. Drugs may not help with a functional disorder, such as irritable bowel syndrome, but diet or stress reduction may help.

Food Allergy and Food Intolerance

Although some people have an unpleasant or dangerous reaction to certain food, that same food may be harmless to others. Peanuts, for example, can be fatal to some. An allergic reaction to food is mediated by the immune system, and it tends to be quite predictable. Each time you eat the food, your symptoms begin very quickly. Intolerance is not allergy, but the two are often confused. An intolerance means a particular food causes your body distress a few hours after you eat it. Many people get diarrhea, cramps, or flatulence from drinking cow's milk. They are not allergic to milk, but their body lacks an enzyme needed to digest the milk sugar lactose.

Food Allergy

Allergies are a reaction of the immune system, but they don't happen on the first exposure to something. It usually shows up on the second or later exposure, once the first contact has sensitized the body to the offending agent. Symptoms of food allergy may include nausea, vomiting, diarrhea, abdominal pain, indigestion, belching, rash, headache, runny nose, hives, asthma, and swelling of the face or throat. True food allergies are rare in adults. In children, however, they are much more common and may be related to the introduction of solid food too soon, before the small intestine has had a chance to mature and produce the needed enzymes. Sometimes the protein in infant formula or cow's milk can cause a reaction.

Foods likely to cause a true allergic reaction in adults are peanuts, milk, eggs, fish (especially shellfish), and wheat. One food allergy involving gluten, a protein found in wheat, can actually damage the cell lining of the small intestine, resulting in poor absorption of nutrients, greasy stools, weight loss, and diarrhea. This is known as gluten-sensitive enteropathy or sprue, nontropical sprue, or celiac disease (see chapter 6).

Food Intolerance

Milk and milk products such as cheese and ice cream are responsible for the most common food intolerance, which affects 30 million to 50 million Americans and millions more around the world. It's the inability to digest lactose, the predominant sugar in milk. Some ethnic populations are more vulnerable than others, especially African Americans, Native Americans, and Mexican Americans. It is least common among people of Northern European descent.

Lactose intolerance comes from a shortage of the enzyme lactase, normally produced by the cells lining the small intestine to break down the milk sugar so it can be absorbed into the bloodstream. Although this condition is not fatal, it can cause nausea, cramps, bloating, gas, and diarrhea. The condition is easily diagnosed with a breath test or stool acidity test (see chapter 11) or careful clinical observation. However, these tests are not 100 percent specific, and in 2003 a new lactose intolerance blood test was made available to identify possible genetic variations responsible for lactose intolerance.

This new test will allow doctors to know if there is a genetic basis for lactose intolerance or if their symptoms are related to another disease or disorder, such as celiac disease or inflammatory bowel disease, which have similar symptoms. Improperly diagnosed and unmanaged, these can lead to serious complications. Until now, diagnostic methods used to detect lactose intolerance could not determine the underlying cause, making treatment choices difficult. The highly specific test identifies patients with a certain genetic marker that is associated with lower-than-normal levels of the lactase enzyme.

There is no cure for lactose intolerance, and avoiding milk sugar is the only treatment. There also are many brands of additives in pill form or chewable tablets that can be used if avoidance of milk and milk products is not practical. Some come as drops you can put into the milk.

Fructose Intolerance

Some people suffer from a more serious problem, known as fructose intolerance or fructose malabsorption, which can be fatal. Technically, it is a hereditary lack of a liver enzyme called aldolase B, which is crucial to the metabolism of fructose, a sugar in soft drinks and juices. To be digested, fructose needs to be broken down before it reaches the colon. If it isn't, it then becomes a high-octane fuel for intestinal bacteria that would otherwise remain docile. This creates hydrogen gas that causes bloating, pain, and loose stools. The undigested fructose collects in the liver and kidneys, and this leads to failure of those organs.

Fructose intolerance occurs more frequently in the United States and northern European countries than anywhere else. One person in every twenty thousand is born with this disorder. When children inherit fructose intolerance from their parents—both parents carry the gene but may not have the condition themselves—it is often hard to diagnose. The baby may become dehydrated, nauseous, and feverish. Loss of appetite and failure to grow are symptoms, and when tremors and seizures occur, they can lead to coma and death.

The condition is diagnosed through urine and blood tests to determine liver and kidney failure. Enzyme studies and a liver biopsy and genetic testing may be called for. The disease can be treated only by completely eliminating fructose and sucrose from the diet. Some people also may need to take medication to lower the level of uric acid in their blood. This will reduce the risk for gout.

Other Reactions to Food

Some people feel pain after eating fatty foods and think they are allergic, but more likely they are suffering from acid reflux or gallstones. Fatty foods tend to relax the lower esophageal sphincter (LES) valve between the stomach and the esophagus, thus creating heartburn. Fatty foods can cause the gallbladder to contract. If gallstones are present, pain results.

Certain foods or their additives and preservatives may cause symptoms that mimic allergies or intolerance but are not. Fermented cheese, pork sausage, canned tuna, and sardines may contain histamine and for some people can cause flushing, headaches, and a drop in blood pressure. Histamine is a chemical the body's immune system makes in response to an allergic reaction. Phenylethylamine, a chemical found in chocolate, red wine, and aged cheese can cause migraine headaches in some people. Monosodium glutamate (MSG) can make a susceptible person dizzy or short of breath. MSG used to be found in great quantities in Chinese food, but many restaurants no longer use it, or, if they do, they say so on the menu. Sulfites often are added to salads and vegetables to preserve a fresh appearance and can cause an asthmatic reaction in some people. Yellow food dye number 5, or tartrazine, found in snacks and drinks, can cause hives, asthma, and a runny nose. Nitrates found in smoked meats and cheese can cause gastrointestinal upset, headache, and hives. Some of these substances affect blood vessels directly, giving rise to flushing, headache, and dizziness.

Lifestyle, Aging, and the Gastrointestinal System

More than twenty thousand pounds of solid foods will be digested by the gastrointestinal tract during your lifetime, so it is a very efficient and hardworking system. The fact that people tend to have problems with their digestive system during or after middle age indicates that it may be affected by wear and tear. Polyps may develop in the colon. Inflammation may develop in the esophagus or the stomach. Valves weaken and ducts get clogged. Think of what happens to your car if it runs for years and many miles without a tune-up. The fuel lines get clogged, sludge forms in the engine, and it doesn't run as efficiently. The digestive system, too, is an energy-driven machine that won't function as well without care.

The digestive system is at our mercy. Some people are born with stronger "constitutions" than others. However, just as the heart is hurt by bad habits such as smoking, a sedentary lifestyle, and poor nutrition, so is the digestive system harmed. And the harm is cumulative as we age.

Everything we eat, drink, or even inhale affects the dynamics of the digestive system. Not only do we get heartburn, bloating, or indigestion, we also can get ulcers, gallstones, constipation, colon polyps—or cancer. Many of these conditions are caused by eating or drinking the wrong foods and liquids, by not exercising enough, and by not understanding how to prevent problems with early intervention or screening.

One of the biggest problems today (no pun intended) is the increasing size of people in the Western world. The numbers of overweight and obese people has caused the American Gastroenterological Association to urge its member physicians to do more about it. Although obesity is not often identified as a gastrointestinal problem, it can certainly lead to problems. The Association is suggesting approaches ranging from portion control to medications, counseling, and group therapy. Doctors believe there would be fewer cases of reflux disease and other digestive complications if people were thinner. Excess abdominal weight puts more pressure on the valve between the esophagus and the stomach, causing acid to back up. Fat accumulations inside the body, especially around the intestines and lining of the abdomen, put pressure on the valve.

When fat cells accumulate in the liver it can cause steatohepatitis (see chapter 9), a condition that leads to dysfunction of the liver. Obesity is strongly associated with gallstones, adult-onset diabetes, and cancer, including cancer of the colon and rectum. Fat will increase the cholesterol in your blood. This not only increases the risk for heart attack and several cancers, but also before it even gets to your blood, it may cause problems. The gallbladder has to process all the fats you eat, and if you overwork that organ, you may develop gallstones.

Fiber in the form of cereals, whole grains, and fresh fruits and vegetables helps flush the fats and waste products from the body with more efficiency. When there is no fiber to transport the waste matter through the colon and out of the body, it stays in the colon where it may contribute to the growth of polyps. These polyps, if undiscovered, can become cancerous. A tendency to constipation may be hereditary, but constipation, more common in women, is frequently felt to be caused by lack of fiber as well as by a sedentary lifestyle. Exercise is critical to bring oxygen to your digestive system and keep the process going, especially through the lower intestinal tract.

Smoking increases your risk of acid reflux disease and esophageal cancer, stomach cancer, and ulcers. These conditions are especially high among smokers, as are cancers of the entire upper digestive tract. You may think the smoke is going only to your lungs, but it is contaminating the upper part of your digestive tract as well—including your mouth.

Drinking too much alcohol is especially harmful. Alcohol is toxic to the stomach lining and other organs, including the liver, where cirrhosis ultimately begins. Excess alcohol is directly responsible for cancer of the esophagus, bleeding of the stomach lining, ulcers, and destruction of the pancreas and liver.

By the time cancer of a digestive organ causes symptoms, it is frequently advanced. Tumors in the system are usually slow-growing, solid tumors and may not be discovered until they have spread outside the digestive tract and caused problems elsewhere.

Systemic Disease Can Cause Digestive Problems

As a review of the contents of any gastroenterology textbook will attest, more than half of the commonly encountered digestive problems are the result of the effect of systemic diseases on the gastrointestinal tract. Here are just a few:

- Atherosclerosis may cause loss of blood (ischemia) to the intestinal tract.
- Abnormally low blood pressure (hypotension) may "shock" the liver and cause hepatitis, from disruption of blood flow and oxygen supply to the liver.
- Diabetes mellitus may cause fatty liver (hepatic steatosis).
- Scleroderma may affect the function of the esophagus and small intestine.
- Stroke may cause difficulty swallowing.
- Toxic amounts of calcium (hypercalcemia) may result in severe constipation.

It is crucial for you and your doctor to recognize and anticipate that some of these conditions will affect your digestive system. Sometimes gastrointestinal symptoms show up before the actual disease, which makes this awareness even more important.

Common Gastrointestinal Symptoms and Problems

The digestive system is complex, and symptoms of many disorders can be similar. Everyone exhibits occasional symptoms, such as gaseousness or nausea, which usually are transitory. However, when these common symptoms become chronic and can't easily be explained, it's time to see your gastroenterologist. Symptoms can be confused with other diseases, too. A spasm in the esophagus can feel just like a heart attack, and to some people it can feel like asthma.

Symptoms that persist or recur should be brought to the attention of your doctor. If you have any of these symptoms, keep a written diary noting any associations with meals, activity, or time of day.

Difficulty Swallowing (Dysphagia)

When it is difficult to swallow solid food and even liquids, you may have esophageal motility problems or an esophageal obstruction. The esophagus can develop problems with the automatic muscular contractions called peristalsis (see pages 72–73). An obstruction, such as a large piece of meat, is called the steakhouse syndrome (see chapter 4). When swallowing is painful, it may indicate inflammation or infection in the esophagus.

Gaseousness and Bloating

Everyone has occasional gas and bloating. Some belching and flatulence is normal. Certain foods produce more gas than others. Gaseousness also is common in people who overeat and in those who are overweight. This can be reduced by eating slowly and chewing food well. If you eliminate chewing gum, smoking, drinking carbonated beverages, and gulping water and other drinks too quickly, you can cut down on the amount of air taken into your digestive system—and thus the amount of air that has to come out one way or another.

Gaseousness and bloating are very nonspecific symptoms and take on meaning only in association with other symptoms.

Noncardiac Chest Pain

Heartburn, indigestion, esophageal spasm, or a gallbladder attack can seem just like a heart attack. This kind of symptom should never be ignored. Your doctor will know how to tell the difference, but sometimes the similarity is so great that tests must be done to rule out a cardiac problem. Any significant chest pain or discomfort (including meal-related) should be considered cardiac until proven otherwise.

Nausea and Vomiting

Many digestive conditions can cause nausea and vomiting, such as a stomach virus, liver disease, or hepatitis. Acute pancreatitis can cause nausea along with knife-like pain in the upper abdomen. Pregnant women often become nauseated in the mornings during their first trimester, but we don't really know why. It may be caused by hormonal changes or lower blood sugar during that period. However, conditions that don't originate in the digestive system, such as dehydration, loss of equilibrium, and vertigo, can cause nausea.

Abdominal Pain

Abdominal pain is a common symptom for a wide variety of gastrointestinal conditions as well as other diseases, such as an ovarian cyst in women. Much abdominal pain can be identified by its location. Pain on the lower left side can be irritable bowel syndrome, diverticulitis, or some other chronic or gynecological problem. On the lower right it could be appendicitis, an ovarian cyst, or Crohn's disease. Pain in the upper abdomen could be caused by the gallbladder, pancreatitis, stomach ulcers, or liver disease. The character of the pain (described to the experienced ears of a physician) can further help define what is going on.

Unexplained Weight Loss

If you are losing weight without trying, it is possible that you have a maldigestion or malabsorption problem. This means your food is not being digested properly and nutrients are not absorbed into the bloodstream. Malabsorption can be a sign of celiac disease. However, this type of weight loss could be a symptom of several other very serious diseases and should never go unreported to your doctor.

Constipation

People can become constipated because of their diet or because they don't drink enough water and get enough exercise. Certain medications also can cause constipation. In addition, it can be caused by blockage in the intestines, or by a class of irritable bowel syndrome. When constipation lasts more than a week it's a good idea to see your doctor. Over-the-counter remedies should be used only occasionally unless you are under the supervision of your doctor.

Diarrhea

Diarrhea can be a temporary result of a stomach virus, food poisoning, or use of certain medications. Many more serious conditions have this symptom, including a class of irritable bowel syndrome, inflammatory bowel disease, Crohn's disease, colon polyps, and celiac disease. If it lasts more than thirty-six hours, call your doctor.

Rectal Bleeding

Blood on the surface of the stool is often caused by hemorrhoids or an anal fissure. Hidden blood in the stool can be a symptom of colon polyps, a tumor, or inflammatory bowel disease. Because you may be unaware of hidden blood, you should discuss with your doctor whether you need a yearly fecal occult blood test (see chapter 2). Never ignore this symptom.

Jaundice

Yellowing of the skin and whites of the eyes is an indication of a liver problem. It could be hepatitis, a blocked bile duct, or cancer of the liver or biliary tree. Jaundice calls for immediate medical attention.

Abdominal Swelling

There is a difference between abdominal bloating and swelling. Bloating is caused by gas and usually is temporary. Swelling can be caused by a collection of fluid in the abdominal space. This is known as ascites and often is a symptom of liver disease. The doctor can feel the water sloshing around on physical exertion.

There are, of course, many other symptoms of digestive diseases, but these are the most common. In the next two chapters you will learn when and how to find a gastroenterologist and what kinds of diagnostic tests (including an entire chapter on endoscopic tests) are available to diagnose symptoms.

Chapter 2

How to Find a Gastroenterologist and the Proper Diagnosis

MEDICINE IS AN EVER-CHANGING science, and this certainly applies to gastroenterology. As a patient you want to have access to the best and latest that modern medicine has to offer. Often this will mean seeing a well-trained gastroenterologist who is board-certified, participates in continuing medical education, and is on the staff of a university teaching hospital or a large suburban hospital.

By finding such a person, it is likely that he or she also will be affiliated with radiologists, surgeons, pathologists, and others who are similarly trained and credentialed. As the field of gastroenterology has evolved, many changes have taken place. Endoscopy has largely replaced barium X-ray studies of the gut. CT, MRI, and sonography have become mainstays of diagnosis of gastrointestinal problems. Endoscopic ultrasound and ERCP (endoscopic retrograde cholangiopancreatography) have become important tools used to diagnose biliary and pancreatic disorders. (Chapter 3 explains endoscopic tests and therapy in detail.)

Capsule camera studies now allow more precise visualization of the small intestine. CT colonography—or virtual colonoscopy—is fast becoming an alternate for conventional endoscopy. New diagnostic blood tests are developed every year. New medications appear monthly. Techniques such as laparoscopic surgery and robotic surgery are becoming the norm. Hospital stays are shortening, and more and more testing and care are being rendered in an outpatient setting. Unfortunately, much of this is being done or developed seemingly at the expense of the doctor-patient-family relationship. We must never lose sight of the dictum *"For the secret of the care of the patient is in caring for the patient."* Francis W. Peabody said this to Harvard students in 1925 in a landmark lecture titled

"The Care of the Patient." His book of the same title is still used in medical schools today.

Most primary care physicians are internists or family practitioners who can treat simple gastrointestinal problems such as indigestion. However, you may need to see a gastroenterologist for persistent discomfort, pain, acid reflux, diarrhea, or constipation. Your primary care physician is not trained to perform endoscopic testing or to interpret many of the newer tests.

A gastroenterologist is an internist who specializes in diagnosis and treatment of diseases of the digestive system and has been trained in endoscopic diagnostic and treatment procedures. In addition to four years of medical school, training includes three to eight years of graduate medical education in the specialty and on-the-job hospital training. The doctor must pass licensing examinations to become accredited.

There are other specialists who treat digestive diseases. A colorectal surgeon has special training in treatment of diseases of the colon, including the rectum and anus. A hepatologist is an internist who limits his or her practice to diseases of the liver, and often has advanced training in gastroenterology as well. An oncologist is an internist who specializes in the treatment of cancer. A radiologist does not evaluate gastrointestinal problems but may be asked to perform diagnostic tests.

A trusting relationship between doctor and patient is essential. Ask other doctors you know for their recommendations. Your primary care physician will be able to recommend one or more gastroenterologists, but it is a good idea to do some research on your own to find a doctor you feel comfortable with. Also talk with patients who have experience with gastroenterologists about how effective their treatment was, and what they liked or disliked about the treatment or the doctor. Many people go from one doctor to another until they find someone who can help them. You should not be reluctant to "doctor-shop" to find the best care possible. Often, people insured with HMOs look in their health care directory and hope for the best. Some are unaware that they can challenge the system and become well-informed patients. If you call your health insurance provider and ask where you can find a doctor who specializes in gastroenterology, they will ask you, "What's your zip code?" They assume that nobody wants to go far from home to find a doctor. Consult more knowledgeable sources such as doctors you know and professional medical associations such as your state medical society; books such as this one; the Internet; and other patients. Ask them what hospitals and doctors have the best reputations for treating your condition.

Your state medical society and the American Medical Association have physician referral services to help you locate a specialist. Go to www.ama-assn.org and click on the AMA Physician Select. Another popular physician listing site is CastleConnolly.com, which has a "Find a Doctor" link. This is a bit like the Zagat ratings of restaurants. Physician profiles are selected after peer nomination, extensive research, and careful review and screening by their own physician-directed research team.

Most states have a department of education that will provide records of the doctor's licensing. To find out if a specialist is accredited, check with the American Board of Medical Specialties. Then you can check with your state department of health to find out if the doctor was subject of any disciplinary action. All of these organizations can be contacted through the Internet. (Keep in mind that there is a great deal of erroneous information on the Internet. For that reason, we've listed some reputable information sources in the back of the book.)

Once your primary care physician learns that you are willing to go to great lengths to get the best care, he or she may help you interpret some of the information you gather. Choose doctors who have not only a great deal of compassion but also up-to-date knowledge and experience and who are able to treat you with the best medical care possible. Once you've found some doctors you believe might be able to help you, talk to them or their office staff before you decide. Many doctors or their office managers will talk with you as a potential patient on the phone for a few minutes if you make an appointment to do this. Be sure to ask about hospital affiliations, hours, availability, and health insurance.

About Diagnostic Testing

There are scores of diagnostic tests for tracking down the cause of digestive diseases. Some, such as breath tests, are easy to do and noninvasive. They can be done by a doctor in the office. Endoscopic tests, on the other hand, require more time and expense. With some, sedatives or anesthesia is needed. They usually involve a technician as well as the doctor, and sometimes more than one doctor (see chapter 3). In another category, scans such as CT or MRI, and the new virtual colonoscopy, require that you go to a medical center or hospital.

Because symptoms are similar for a variety of gastroenterological conditions, most diagnoses must be made through a process of excluding all possibilities. Before any diagnostic tests are performed, a physical examination as well as a detailed history of symptoms and lifestyle are needed.

Since the 1970s it has become much easier to look inside the digestive system to find out what exactly is wrong. Endoscopic procedures usually are more expensive than regular X-rays, but they are the most effective. In the past (and still today) barium enemas were given as an X-ray examination to look inside the colon. Colonoscopy is much more efficient, but as we will see later, there are certain instances where a barium enema X-ray is still recommended. Such tests should be done only by a qualified and experienced physician, and they should be done where there is access to the most up-to-date equipment.

Noninvasive Tests

Breath tests, stool tests, blood tests, and simple X-rays can be used to find out if the problem can be solved quickly or if more testing is needed to pinpoint diagnosis.

Breath Tests

A breath test is a simple, quick, and safe way to investigate several digestive diseases before doing more invasive tests. Both the hydrogen breath tests and the new 13C stable radioisotope breath tests are nonradioactive and safe for anyone, including children and pregnant women. Breath tests can help identify *Helicobacter pylori* infection, bacterial overgrowth, bile salt waste, lactose and fructose intolerance, and pancreatic insufficiency.

Normally there is no hydrogen in the breath. But let's say you are lactose-intolerant. Undigested lactose forms gases, including hydrogen, in the colon. The hydrogen is absorbed from the intestines and carried through the bloodstream to the lungs and exhaled. To take the test you drink a lactose-loaded beverage, and then your exhaled breath is analyzed at regular intervals.

In another example, the *H. pylori* bacteria in the stomach can convert a naturally occurring substance called urea into carbon dioxide, ammonia, and water. If you swallow a special solution and then exhale, the test can identify that. A tiny amount of non radioactive-labeled urea is put into a glass of orange juice that you drink. Half an hour later, you blow into a small test tube. If *H. pylori* is present in the stomach, it will digest the urea and release a small amount of the tracer with the breath. This safe and easy test is more accurate than a blood test. It can detect active infection, whereas the blood test can tell only if you had been exposed to *H. pylori* at some time in life and developed antibodies. Breath tests also are very useful in checking on whether an infection has been successfully treated.

Fasting is required the night before this test, and you need to talk with your doctor about medications you need to stop taking ahead of time. Accuracy of the breath test is reduced if you have been taking certain drugs, such as antibiotics, during the previous weeks.

Blood Tests

Several blood tests can be used to track various digestive diseases. A complete blood count (CBC) tests for anemia, which can result from blood loss from the gut. In addition, blood tests can be targeted at liver enzymes, bilirubin and bile salt levels, hepatitis, pancreatitis, malabsorption, and inflammation. Some are designed to monitor treatment with medications, identify people with inflammatory blood disease, help differentiate Crohn's disease from ulcerative colitis, identify liver fibrosis in people with hepatitis C, identify gluten sensitivity, and find out if certain medications would be toxic to some people.

Stool Acidity Test

The stool acidity test is often used to measure the amount of acid in the stool of infants and young children to determine if they are lactose-intolerant. Undigested lactose is fermented by bacteria in the colon and creates lactic acid and fatty acids that can be found in stool samples. Glucose also may be present in the sample because it is not being absorbed by the colon.

Fecal Occult Blood Test

The loss of blood that is hidden in the stool can indicate ulcers or polyps and is the most common sign of cancer of the colon and rectum. The fecal occult blood test, first introduced to clinical practice in the 1950s, has come to be regarded as a valuable aid in colorectal and gastrointestinal cancer surveillance.

The fecal occult blood test (FOBT) is a simple test using a card on which samples of stool can be smeared and analyzed. The currently available guaiac-impregnated cards are very accurate when used properly. These cards are most often given to patients by their physicians, but FOBT cards are often available at hospital and health fairs (such as those in communities or malls), and from nurses or health offices in the workplace. And, like the home pregnancy test, the FOBT also is available over the counter in some drugstores.

The collection of two smears per day from different parts of the stool for three days is recommended. A chemical is applied to the samples at the doctor's office or at a laboratory, or a person can do it at home. If the sample turns blue, it indicates the presence of blood in the stool.

Before testing for hidden blood, patients often are asked to follow a special diet for two days because the digestion of certain foods can cause a false positive or false negative result. (Patients do not always comply with these dietary restrictions, and some do not supply the number of samples required.) For example, fiber is allowed because it is believed to stimulate bleeding from any existing polyps protruding into the colon passageway. On the other hand, aspirin is to be avoided because it can cause bleeding that has nothing to do with a possible polyp in the colon, and it could cause a false positive result.

Other foods and substances to avoid for that reason include red meat, turnips, horseradish, citrus fruits and vitamin C, and iron supplements. Patients are asked to eat high-fiber foods such as bran, peanuts, and popcorn, as well as fruits and vegetables, chicken, and tuna fish.

Absorption Tests

Several tests can be used to find out why the digestive system is not properly absorbing nutrients from food.

D-Xylose Absorption Test

Lower-than-normal amounts of D-xylose in the blood and urine samples may suggest that the small intestine is not absorbing nutrients from food properly. This could be caused by Crohn's disease, sprue, or celiac disease. It also may indicate inflammation in the lining of the small intestine from an infection or from a parasite, such as giardiasis or hookworm.

For this test, a drink containing sugar is swallowed, and later urine and blood are tested for levels of D-xylose, a type of sugar normally absorbed by the intestine but not used in the body. This is a test to determine if the intestine is absorbing nutrients properly. If it is not, the amounts of D-xylose in the blood and urine will be low.

Before the test there must be abstinence from foods and liquids high in pentose, a sugar similar to D-xylose. These include fruits, jams, and pastries. Some medications also may interfere with the test, so your doctor may stop these temporarily before the test. Urine is checked before the test and then after drinking a solution with D-xylose. Then blood samples are collected within two hours of taking the solution and again five hours later. All of the urine produced over the five-hour period also will be collected and tested. Sometimes this urine collection is extended for twenty-four hours.

Schilling Test for B_{12} Absorption

Deficiency of vitamin B_{12} is often an indication of anemia, gastric atrophy, bacterial overgrowth, or disease of the ileum. This test can identify the deficiency.

Serum Carotene Levels

Carotene is a fat-soluble substance found in yellow vegetables and fruits as well as in eggs. Serum carotene levels tend to be depressed in patients who don't absorb fats. However, they also can be depressed if intake of dietary carotene is low.

Stool Test for Fecal Fat

When too much fat is detected in stool, it means it is not being absorbed properly in the digestive system. This could be due to failure of the bile system, severe liver disease, or bacterial overgrowth in the small intestine. The test can evaluate how fats are digested by determining if there is excessive excretion of lipids in people who show signs of malabsorption such as weight loss, abdominal distention, and scaly skin.

Stool must be collected over a seventy-two-hour period while the patient maintains a high-fat diet. Alcohol and certain drugs must be withheld during this time because they can affect the results.

Electrogastrogram

An electrogastrogram (EGG) is like an electrocardiogram (EKG) of the heart. It records electrical signals that travel through the muscles of the stomach and control the reaction of those muscles. The EGG is used to confirm a doctor's suspicion that the stomach muscles or the nerves controlling them are not working normally.

Electrodes are taped over the abdomen, and the sounds are recorded on a computer. The test, which takes about three hours, usually is done after fasting and then again after eating. Normally there is a regular rhythm generated by the stomach muscles, just like there is in the heart. The power—electrical voltage—increases after a meal. When there are abnormalities in those muscles or nerves, the rhythm is often irregular, or there is no increase after eating.

There is no other test like this one, but antroduodenal motility studies or gastric emptying studies may provide additional information. Abnormal electrical activity of the stomach sometimes results in abnormal muscular activity and reduced emptying of food from the stomach.

The EGG is still considered an experimental procedure, and its exact role in diagnosis of stomach disease is not yet defined.

Abdominal Sonography

Abdominal ultrasound is used to image the liver, gallbladder, spleen, pancreas, and kidneys. The blood vessels of these organs also can be evaluated. Ultrasound sends out high-frequency sound waves that reflect off body structures to create a picture. There is no radiation exposure with this test. This also can be done endoscopically (see chapter 3). Ultrasound sometimes is used to supplement endoscopy to determine if a lesion is solid. The physician or a technician scans your abdomen by a handheld transducer or probe that converts the sound waves that bounce off your body into images on a screen.

Radiological Tests

When simple tests are not conclusive, then X-rays and other radiological tests such CT scans are needed to see images inside the body.

Barium X-rays, Upper GI Series

Also called barium swallows and upper GI series, this is done when endoscopy cannot be used, when there is difficulty swallowing, or ulcer symptoms, heartburn, or occult gastrointestinal bleeding. It can help diagnose narrowing of the esophagus, inflammation or strictures of the esophagus, hiatal hernia, spasms, and gastric and duodenal ulcers or tumors.

Barium is a radiopaque liquid that shows up white in X-rays. After you swallow it, a radiologist uses a fluoroscope connected to a TV monitor to observe the progress of barium through your digestive tract. The radiologist takes a series of X-rays of the esophagus, stomach, and the first part of the small intestine (duodenum). If Crohn's disease is suspected, a similar test will be performed immediately afterward to examine the entire length—more than twenty feet—of the small intestine. Sometimes the procedure uses "double contrast" media. This means you also swallow tablets to release gas in your stomach. The gas helps to show the stomach lining in greater detail.

Barium Enema X-ray

This X-ray procedure sometimes is used in conjunction with sigmoid-oscopy to provide complementary information, especially if an obstruction is detected in the colon. The barium enema X-ray is still a time-honored tool for finding polyps, but not all physicians find it necessary. Most believe that if a polyp is found with sigmoidoscopy, then the patient should proceed to the more accurate colonoscopy to examine the entire length of the colon and should have the polyp removed and a biopsy done at the same time. However, some health insurance companies and health maintenance organizations might require the barium enema X-ray as part of the screening procedure for colon cancer because it is generally less expensive than colonoscopy.

After the colon is cleansed with enemas, an inert substance containing barium is inserted into the rectum and colon through the anus. Barium appears opaque on X-rays. The camera watches under fluoroscopic guidance and X-ray pictures as the barium fills the colon and rectum. To make small tumors easier to see, the doctor also might expand the colon by carefully pumping in air during the test. This is called an air contrast or double contrast barium enema and improves the accuracy of the standard barium enema X-ray.

A technician generally performs a large part of the procedure in conjunction with a physician (radiologist). The physician will look at the films as they are developed and possibly again later. The sensitivity of this screening procedure is directly related to the patience and diligence of the technician and physician performing the procedure. Overlapping loops of bowel can be difficult to interpret, and extensive diverticulosis or residual fecal material also can interfere with an accurate reading. There is normally a small risk associated with radiation exposure, but the real limitation in this procedure is that a biopsy or polypectomy cannot be performed if a polyp is discovered. The test takes about an hour.

After the test you'll need to drink plenty of fluids and rest. The procedure can be tiring. Also, you may need to take another enema to rid the colon of any remaining barium. You may have pale-colored stools for the next day or two.

Abdominal X-ray

An abdominal X-ray is helpful in ruling out free air within the abdominal cavity; this air shows up just under the diaphragm and if present could indicate a ruptured bowel or appendix. The air pattern within the intestinal tract is useful in diagnosis. Usually air is seen in the loops of the large intestine. When air is prominent in the small intestine or the stomach, intestinal obstruction is likely. Occasionally a kidney stone, gallstone, or pancreatic calcification can be visualized on X-ray.

Be sure to inform your doctor if you are pregnant or have an IUD inserted, or if you have had a barium-contrast X-ray in the previous four days. Also, if you have taken medications such as Pepto-Bismol (which contains bismuth) within four days, let the doctor know because it could interfere with the test.

Oral Cholecystogram

This is a test to get images of the gallbladder and is performed in a hospital radiology department or freestanding radiology facility. The night before the test, you are asked to swallow some pills that contain the contrast medium that allows visualization of the gallbladder during the X-ray. Then you can eat a fat-free meal. However, once the tablets have been ingested, you cannot drink any liquid. The doctor uses a fluoroscope, a special X-ray that projects images onto a video monitor. You may be asked to assume various positions. Additionally, you may be asked to drink a high-fat formula that will force the gallbladder to contract and release some bile.

Computerized Tomographic Scan

A computerized tomographic (CT) scan is an excellent way to look at the abdominal wall and the lymph-node-bearing areas of the abdomen, liver, and other solid organs for signs of cancer metastasis. While you lie inside a wide tube, this X-ray translates information into two-dimensional "slices," or cross sections. The radiation dose from a CT scan is considerably higher than from a routine X-ray. The amount depends on the number of slices needed and on the part of the body. A CT scan also is used in planning radiation treatment to outline the field or area to be treated. A CT scan offers the best initial evaluation of the pancreas and is 85 percent specific in chronic pancreatitis. CT provides good visualization of the entire liver and pancreas to spot any complications. It also is used for diagnosing diverticulitis. A CT scan can be done to the entire body or particular areas.

If your doctor has asked for a contrast-enhanced CT scan, you will be injected with a contrast agent and X-rays will be taken. It is important to remain very still during the scanning so the X-rays will not be blurred. CT scans are a hundred times more sensitive than regular X-rays and can allow the radiologist to see minute differences in soft tissue within the body.

Helical or spiral CT of the abdomen and pelvis requires fasting for four to six hours if contrast dye is to be used or sedation is anticipated.

CT Colonography (Virtual Colonoscopy)

Virtual colonoscopy is an examination of the colon without an invasive tube. It combines X-rays and computers to view inside the entire colon without inserting anything but air. This is a relatively new form of X-ray technology called spiral CT. The exam takes ten to twenty minutes and requires no sedation. It is less expensive than conventional colonoscopy.

Virtual colonoscopy is now being performed at more and more medical centers and gastroenterology diagnostic centers. It does the same thing a colonoscopy does but without the discomfort or the expense. This newly developed technique uses a CT scanner and computer virtual reality software to see inside the colon without using the long endoscopic tube. Virtual colonoscopy is better able to detect polyps than a barium enema and is almost as accurate as conventional colonoscopy. It is useful for very frail patients or if a large tumor blocks the passage through the colon.

The procedure begins with a standard CT scan of the abdomen. This allows radiologists to create pictures on the computer that look like those seen by the conventional colonoscope. Preparation is similar—that is, you need to take the cleansing lavage the day before the procedure and come into the test with a clean bowel (see chapter 3). A small flexible rubber is placed in the rectum, but this is only to introduce air into the colon. This may cause minor gas pain or abdominal cramping. If it's too uncomfortable, the doctor can give you a medication to relax the colon. You lie on your back and then on your stomach, and the total procedure is done in ten to twenty minutes. Because no sedation is necessary, you can resume normal activity immediately after the test.

The disadvantages compared to conventional colonoscopy are that it offers less detail of the inside of the colon, and the images are in black and white. This lack of color makes it more difficult to evaluate lesions. Also, small polyps are less likely to be located, even though conventional colonoscopy still misses as much as 20 percent of them and up to 5 percent of colon cancers. Most insurance companies do not cover CT colonography as a screening test for polyps, but some may cover it for people who already have symptoms of colon disease.

Magnetic Resonance Imaging

Like a CT scan, magnetic resonance imaging (MRI) can give a better image of the solid abdominal organs and lymph nodes than that obtained by the other methods. Scientists are developing the MRI capability to differentiate between malignant and benign processes and to evaluate lymph nodes for metastasis. Patients often are afraid of the procedure because it means being confined in a long tube for as long as an hour. However, a mild sedative makes most claustrophobic patients relax. At some diagnostic centers, open-air MRI is becoming available. However, this may not be as accurate.

A number of gastrointestinal disorders lend themselves to investigation with MRI: liver, pancreas, spleen, gallbladder, and biliary tract. Ordinarily there is no preparation necessary for an MRI.

Magnetic Resonance Cholangiopancreatography

Cholangiopancreatography is an MRI of the abdomen and pelvis. Magnetic resonance cholangiopancreatography MRCP is a noninvasive method for evaluating the biliary tract ductal system around the liver, pancreas, and gallbladder. It is especially good for spotting possible tumors in the biliary tree and provides good visualization of ducts, with clarity similar to the invasive ERCP (see chapter 3). This test may precede an ERCP in people with low likelihood of intervention. MRCP is similar to MRI but you cannot eat or drink for at least three hours before the procedure. This ensures high-quality pictures.

Angiogram

A coronary angiogram is called for if symptoms of heartburn or similar digestive problems could be confused with heart disease. The test would be used to rule out any coronary disease. An angiogram is an X-ray of the arteries on the surface of the heart. It allows the doctor to see if any of those arteries are blocked with plaque. An angiogram is one of the most accurate tests for diagnosing coronary artery disease.

To do this test, the physician injects a contrast medium into the coronary arteries via a catheter. Usually this is done by inserting the catheter through a blood vessel in the upper thigh and moving the catheter all the way up to the heart. Once in place, the catheter serves as a vessel through which to inject the dye into the arteries so the X-ray can be taken.

You are awake for this procedure, but the area around the thigh will be numbed and you'll get a mild sedative. Ordinarily you won't feel any movement of the catheter.

Because an artery is punctured for an angiogram, there is risk involved. Rarely, internal bleeding or hemorrhage may occur. Also, if there is a blood clot or plaque in the artery, the angiogram may dislodge it and trigger a stroke or a heart attack. The contrast dye also may cause allergic reactions. Because of such risks, an angiogram usually is done in the hospital during an overnight stay so the patient can be watched after the procedure.

Abdominal MR Angiogram

Instead of angiography, three-dimensional magnetic resonance angiography is used to evaluate diseases of the abdominal aorta, the main artery going from the heart to the body. This is a highly accurate technique to evaluate aortic aneurysms. It is safe and fast and less expensive than conventional angiography. The exam takes about thirty minutes. Similarly, the abdominal aortic angiogram allows the doctor to look at the abdominal aorta.

Celiac and Mesenteric Angiography

The celiac and mesenteric arteries and branches of the abdominal aorta can be explored with this type of X-ray. It is commonly used to detect aneurysm, thrombosis, and signs of ischemia and to locate the source of gastrointestinal bleeding. It is used to diagnose cirrhosis. The procedure can take up to three hours depending on how many blood vessels are studied.

Splenoportography

This variation of an angiogram involves injecting a contrast dye directly into the spleen to view the veins. It can diagnose blockages in those veins and also is used to assess the strength of the area's vascular system before liver transplantation.

Nuclear Scans

When you get an X-ray or a CT scan, the radiation comes from a machine and passes through your body. A nuclear scan works the opposite way. The radiation comes from your body (where it has been injected) and is then detected by a gamma camera. While X-rays can tell us what an organ looks like, nuclear scans tell us how the organ functions. They can see what part of the organ is working properly—or not. In this way an infection or an invasion by a tumor can be seen weeks or months before any abnormality would show up on X-rays or a CT scan.

Nuclear scans are safe and painless. A small amount of radioactive material, known as a tracer, is introduced into the body by injection, or by swallowing or inhalation. The camera follows the tracer in the organ or tissue being imaged and records the data on a computer screen. Nuclear scans carry about the same risk as an X-ray. The tracer loses its radioactivity in a few hours, and the material passes out of the body within a day.

The only people who should not get such a scan are pregnant women and children.

HIDA Scan

A cholescintigraphy (HIDA) scan is done by nuclear medicine physicians to diagnose obstruction of the bile ducts by a gallstone or a tumor, disease of the gallbladder, and bile leaks. It also is called a hepatobiliary scan or radionucleide scan. It diagnoses abnormal contraction of the gallbladder or an obstruction. It can be used when ultrasound doesn't provide enough visualization in cases of poor liver function, cancer, or an abscess in the area. Overall, it may be the most sensitive test for acute cholecystitis. It also works with people who have had prior gallbladder surgery, or poor gallbladder emptying, and those who have eaten just before the test.

A radioactive agent called a bile tracer is injected intravenously into the patient. This test chemical is removed from the blood by the liver and secreted into the bile produced by the liver. The chemical goes anywhere the bile goes—into the ducts, gallbladder, and intestines—while a camera follows it. The camera that senses radioactivity is placed over the abdomen and gets pictures of the liver bile ducts and gallbladder. The test takes about two hours.

Various patterns of the radioactive chemical trail help form a diagnosis. If the chemical is not detected in the liver, a diseased liver is probably the reason. If the chemical is absorbed by the liver but not secreted into the bile ducts, there probably is an obstruction of the ducts exiting the liver. When it fails to show up in the gallbladder but is detected in the intestine, there is an obstruction of the cystic duct leading to and from the gallbladder. If the chemical appears outside the liver, ducts, gallbladder, and intestine, there probably is a bile leak from the ducts or gallbladder.

Cholescintigraphy is most commonly used to diagnose gallbladder problems when other tests are normal. The test can be modified to watch the gallbladder contract and squeeze out its bile. This test does not work on anyone with elevated bilirubin levels.

Liver and Spleen Scan

This test is the best way to study the liver without surgery. The scan uses a radioactive isotope to evaluate liver and/or spleen function. The isotope is injected into a vein, and after the isotope has had time to be absorbed into the bloodstream, the patient lies under a scanner. The liver and spleen should appear normal in shape, location, and size. There is no pain in this test, but if you are tense, you may need a sedative. Abnormal results could indicate liver disease, abscess, infection, cancer, or a number of other conditions. Other tests, such as CT scan or ultrasound, may be needed to confirm results of this scan.

Red Blood Cell Nuclear Scan

A red blood cell (RBC) nuclear scan can find the site of gastrointestinal bleeding. A sample of your blood is drawn and mixed with a tiny amount of radioactive material and re-injected back into your body. While you lie on your back on a table, a camera-like machine above takes pictures of your abdomen for two hours. In addition to locating the site of bleeding in the GI tract, this test is sometimes used to evaluate the rate of blood loss in some cases of anemia, to evaluate blood vessel obstructions, or to look for a hemangioma within the liver.

The exposure to radiation is minimal from the radioisotope that decomposes and is gone within twelve hours. Nevertheless, this test is not recommended for pregnant or nursing women.

Positron Emission Tomography (PET)

Positron emission tomography (PET) scans are used for diagnosing brain, heart, and many other conditions, including cancer. This scan can help pinpoint the source of cancer, and we know that if most cancers are caught early, they can be cured. A CT or MRI cannot detect active tumors. A scan of the entire body can help doctors find out if the cancer has spread to other organs. Cancer cells are highly metabolic, and they synthesize the radioactive glucose (sugar) that is injected into the patient before the scan. Areas of high glucose intake are displayed quite clearly in the scan imagery. The radioactive material injected is no greater than for most other nuclear scans.

At present PET scans have only limited applicability to gastrointestinal problems.

Diagnostic testing also includes biopsy, but these tests are included in chapters on specific gastrointestinal conditions.

Chapter 3

What You Need to Know about Endoscopic Procedures for Diagnosis and Treatment

SINCE THE 1970S, it has become much easier to look inside the digestive system and find out what exactly is wrong. Endoscopic procedures usually are more expensive than regular X-rays and other scans but are the most effective. In the past (and still to some extent today) barium enema X-ray examinations were given before a decision was made to look inside the colon with the more invasive colonoscopy. Endoscopic colonoscopy is much more efficient. However, such tests should be done only by a trained gastroenterologist-endoscopist, and they should be done where there is access to the most up-to-date equipment.

Most primary care physicians are not trained in the use of endoscopic procedures and will refer you to a gastroenterologist or surgeon specially trained in this procedure. As part of their education, gastroenterologists receive extensive endoscopic training in performing colonoscopy, polypectomy, and biopsy thoroughly, safely, and with a minimum amount of patient discomfort. Some surgeons also receive this training, particularly if they are surgical subspecialists such as colorectal surgeons.

Many studies have shown that patients are at much higher risk of serious injury or death when a delicate procedure or surgery is done by a doctor or surgeon who does not do the procedure very often. In 2003, new information was released by the Center for Medical Consumers that confirmed earlier studies. In 1998 a study found that when a carotid endarterectomy was performed by a surgeon who did fewer than five a year at a hospital that did fewer than a hundred a year, the death rate was more than twice as high as when the doctor and the hospital did it more frequently. There were similar findings for other procedures. Though most colonoscopies were done by doctors who did several hundred each in 2001, almost half the doctors did only one.

An endoscope is a tube with a tiny light and a camera that can travel into the digestive system from the mouth or from the anus and send images back to a video screen monitored by the doctor. The risk of getting an infection from an endoscope is very low. After each procedure an endoscope is put through rigorous cleansing and sterilizing treatments designed by the American Society for Gastrointestinal Endoscopy. If you are allergic to latex, be sure to let your doctor know ahead of time. The procedure then needs to be done in a latex-free environment.

Endoscopy is used for diagnosis and treatment. For example, if a polyp is discovered in the colon during a colonoscopy, it can be removed.

Questions to Ask before You Get an Endoscopic Procedure

There are certain endoscopic standards recognized by the American Society of Gastrointestinal Endoscopy (ASGE) that can help you make your choice. Before you consent to having an endoscopic procedure, ask the following questions:

1. Where did the physician receive his or her training in endoscopy? A gastroenterologist is trained in endoscopy by other physicians as part of his or her postgraduate medical training. Ask about the doctor's training before you get ready for the procedure, not the minute before the endoscope is to be inserted into your body.

2. Will the procedure by monitored by video? This is recommended because you (and your doctor) can retain hard-copy pictures of the procedure.

3. Do the physicians and technicians performing endoscopic procedures observe standard precautions? They should abide by these precautions and wear gloves, masks, and gowns during the procedure.

4. Will a biopsy be done? A biopsy is standard practice whenever a polyp or a piece of tissue is removed from the digestive tract.

5. Where and by whom will the biopsy be examined? Ask about the pathologist and the pathology laboratory. Find out if the pathology will be done in the same medical center or sent to another lab.

You might check this with your insurance company as well, to make sure they cover the particular pathology lab.

6. How long will it take for the pathology report? For the procedure report? Usually it takes about four business days to find out the results. Ask for an estimated time to call for results. Understand that if this takes longer, it does not necessarily mean the results are bad; it only means your anxiety level is higher. Sometimes there are delays in hospitals and labs.

7. Will you be given conscious sedation with medications such as Demerol, Diprivan, Valium, or Versed? And who will give you the anesthesia if it is used? Sometimes an anesthetist is required to administer these substances, and sometimes the gastroenterologist can do it. This depends on the regulations of the particular diagnostic center. In any case, you will need a friend or family member to take you home if you are sedated.

8. Who will be present during the procedure? Generally, a gastroenterologist does the procedure with the help of an assistant, who may be a technician or a physician's assistant or nurse. An anesthesiologist may be present to render conscious sedation.

9. What will it cost, and what does the cost include?

To find a medical center with proper endoscopic standards in your area, you also can call one of the cancer information hotlines listed in the appendix or check local health networks. The ASGE can help you locate a gastrointestinal endoscopist through their Web site at www.asge.org. Click on "Find an Endoscopist." They also provide information on various endoscopic procedures.

Manometry (Motility) Tests

Manometry is a technique for measuring squeeze pressures in various parts of the intestine. It uses long, thin tubes through which pressure wave forms can be recorded. Gastroenterologists have lots of information about normal pressure wave forms in the digestive system, so manometric testing easily identifies abnormalities. The method of testing varies according to which part of the intestine is being studied.

Esophageal Manometry

The esophagus has a sphincter at the upper and lower ends. During an esophageal manometry test, the function of the sphincters as well as the tubular esophagus are tested. Often this is done when somebody has difficulty swallowing and tests show no blockage. It is the best test when achalasia is suspected (see chapter 4). It also is helpful in documenting problems with the sphincters and esophageal contraction. Esophageal manometry usually is done on people with severe gastrointestinal reflux disease (GERD) before surgery is done to repair a hiatal hernia. Eight hours of fasting are required before the test. The tube is passed through the nose after a local anesthetic is applied to the throat and is done while you are lying down. Then you are asked to breathe in and out and swallow small sips of water while the doctor watches on the computer screen.

In addition to achalasia, this test detects esophageal abnormalities such as nutcracker esophagus, diffuse esophageal spasm, scleroderma esophagus, and nonspecific motor disorders that cause trouble swallowing or chest pain.

Gastroduodenal Manometry

This tests pressure changes within the stomach and upper intestine during digestion. It is similar to esophageal manometry but takes longer and requires more sedation because the tube is manipulated while it is watched with X-ray. The tube is inserted and removed through the nose.

Anorectal Manometry

This test measures the pressure of the anal sphincter muscles. It also measures how well somebody can feel different sensations of fullness in the rectum. Preparation for this test involves a self-administered cleansing enema that can be purchased in a drugstore. Four hours of fasting also are required before the test. An endoscopic tube is inserted through the anus as a small amount of water drips into the tube from an attached machine. This machine measures pressure. The patient is asked to squeeze the rectal muscles, relax, and push. The muscles and sphincter in this area are tested when someone has incontinence or constipation.

Upper Endoscopy: Esophagogastroduodenoscopy

An upper GI endoscopy provides a thorough examination of the esophagus, stomach, and duodenum. This testing will detect abnormalities in the mucous membrane, cellular changes, Barrett's metaplasia, or any other complications. The video camera allows the doctor to see inflammation or irritation of the tissue lining the esophagus (esophagitis). If the findings are abnormal or questionable, a biopsy can be done by removing a piece of tissue. This test should be considered if you have poorly controlled reflux symptoms, particularly if you are over fifty.

Before the procedure it is necessary to fast so there is no food in your esophagus or stomach. The back of your throat is numbed by a local anesthetic, and a sedative will relax you.

Esophageal dilation is a procedure that dilates or stretches a narrowed area of the esophagus. As a treatment, it may be done several times for gradual expansion. It also is sometimes used as a diagnostic tool along with upper endoscopy to detect problems inside the esophagus. (See the next section for more detail on how this procedure is used in treatment.)

Esophageal pH Probe

A pH probe of the esophagus is the gold standard diagnostic test for reflux disease. By monitoring you for twenty-four-hour periods, your doctor can determine the acidity level of your esophagus and how your symptoms change during meals, activity, and sleep. When a symptom such as chest pain correlates on a temporal basis with a drop in the pH of the esophagus, the pain is caused by acid reflux. Newer techniques of long-term pH monitoring are improving diagnostic capability.

The esophageal pH test measures how often stomach acid flows into the lower esophagus. A small probe at the end of a tube does the measuring. The tube is gently inserted through the nose to reach the end of the esophagus. It is attached to a small portable recorder you carry at your waist for twenty-four hours. Whenever you experience reflux or other symptoms, you press a button on the recorder to mark the time. Later, when reading the printout from the recorder, the doctor will be able to note the acidity level at each marked time.

Eight hours before you begin this test, you must abstain from food or liquid. This is so your doctor can examine the esophagus in its natural state. Any medications that affect the acid flow are usually discontinued at least forty-eight hours before the test, as are caffeine and alcohol.

It takes less than fifteen minutes to place the pH probe while you sit on a chair or lie on your side. As you swallow, the tip of the tube enters the esophagus and the medical technician or doctor passes it to the target area. You may gag slightly, but this is easily controlled. Once the tube is taped to your nose and connected to the recording device, it's well tolerated.

The tube is sensitive to changes in acid concentration. Sometimes two sensors are used if trying to determine if breathing problems or hoarseness is caused by acid reflux. You will be given a diary in which to record anything that affects reflux, such as eating or changing your position. When the tube is removed, the data from the recording device are downloaded into a computer.

Endoscopic Retrograde Cholangiopancreatography

This is a combination of endoscopy and radiography that allows visualization of the biliary ductal pattern from the liver and pancreas, and changes caused by inflammation or tumors. Endoscopic retrograde cholangiopancreatography (ERCP) is the gold standard for getting a close look at a pancreas with chronic disease. A special side-viewing endoscope is passed through the mouth into the digestive tract, and the tip is placed in the duodenum. This is the first portion of the small intestine where the common bile duct and pancreatic duct empty through a valve called the sphincter of Oddi.

ERCP must be done on an empty stomach, so for six hours before the procedure you cannot eat. Your doctor may want you to refrain from certain medications as well. During this procedure, which takes place on an X-ray table, you are sedated intravenously. Sometimes antibiotics also are given before the procedure. Once the endoscope is in place, a catheter connected to a syringe with radiopaque dye is inserted through it. The tip of the catheter is threaded through the sphincter into the common bile duct and/or the pancreatic duct. The dye is injected, and X-rays are taken to show the ducts. This is how we look for duct stones, chronic pancreatitis, and cancers of the bile duct and pancreas. During ERCP a tissue sample can be removed for a biopsy. There may be some discomfort when the doctor blows air into the duodenum and injects the dye into the ducts. However, the sedative and pain medication will reduce the discomfort.

When the sedative wears off you can go home, but some patients may need to stay in the hospital for a day. Possible complications of ERCP include pancreatitis, infection, bleeding, and perforation of the duodenum. Except for pancreatitis, these problems are rare. ERCP takes from thirty minutes to two hours.

ERCP can treat problems as well as detect them. Stones can be extracted from the ducts. Blocked ducts can be reopened by placing another special tube, a stent, through the obstruction. Scars and leaks (from trauma or surgery) and cancer also can be treated. Treatments with ERCP include the following:

Sphincterotomy   This involves cutting the muscle that surrounds the opening of the ducts to enlarge the opening. This is done while the doctor looks through the ERCP scope at the duct opening. A small wire on a specialized catheter uses electric current to cut the tissue. There is no discomfort because there are no nerve endings there. The actual cut is quite small, usually less than half an inch, but it allows various treatments in the ducts. Most commonly the cut is directed toward the bile duct, called a biliary sphincterotomy. Sometimes the cut is directed toward the pancreatic duct, depending on the type of treatment you need.

Stone removal   This is the most common treatment through an ERCP scope. Bile duct stones may have formed in the gallbladder and traveled into the bile duct, or they may form in the duct itself years after the gall-bladder has been removed. A sphincterotomy enlarges the opening of the duct so stones can be pulled from the duct into the bowel. A variety of balloons and baskets attached to specialized catheters can be passed through the ERCP scope into the ducts. Very large stones may need crushing in the duct with a special basket so the fragments can be pulled out during the spincterotomy.

Stent placement   This is done into the bile or pancreatic duct to bypass strictures, the narrowed areas of the duct caused by scar tissue or tumors blocking normal drainage. Two types of stents are commonly used. One looks like a small plastic straw. This type is pushed through the ERCP scope into the blocked duct so it can drain. The other type is made of metal wires resembling the cross wires of a fence. The metal stent is flex-ible and springs open to become wider than the straw type. Both types of stent tend to clog up after several months and may need to be replaced. Metal stents are permanent, while plastic stents are easily removed.

Balloon dilation   This is used to stretch out a narrow opening. ERCP catheters are fitted with dilating balloons, which are then inflated. Often this is performed when the cause of the narrowing is benign. After bal-loon dilation, a stent may be placed for several months to help maintain the dilation.

Flexible Sigmoidoscopy

There has been a significant reduction in colon cancer deaths because of the increase in diagnostic screening sigmoidoscopy. Even one screening in a ten-year period reduced the risk by 79 percent, according to a study at the University of Wisconsin. Approximately two-thirds of colon polyps are within reach of the flexible fiberoptic proctosigmoidoscope. This instrument, about 1.5 to 2 feet long, sends a tiny video camera into the sigmoid area, or left side of the colon. This instrument is widely used today, replacing the more objectionable rigid instruments in use until the 1970s. This older technique is far from ideal for screening purposes. It is unpopular with patients and physicians and provides consistent examination of only the lower 60 centimeters, about 24 inches, of the colon and rectum.

If you are preparing for a flexible sigmoidoscopy, which can be done in your gastroenterologist's office or the endoscopy suite of a hospital, your doctor might have you self-administer two enemas at home the night before. (An enema is the insertion of fluid into the rectum through the anus, which causes the evacuation of fecal matter from the rectum.) Some doctors prescribe a gentle overnight laxative preparation. You will be asked to refrain from eating after midnight and to come to the procedure with an empty colon. No sedation is necessary for this procedure, but you might occasionally feel some pressure, like a gas pain.

While you lie on your side, the endoscopist manipulates the scope through your colon. If you are curious, you can watch the progress of the scope on the video monitor with your physician. The colon is flexible, with many loops and folds, and appears pink on the video monitor.

When a polyp is found during a sigmoidoscopy, it is customary to recommend colonoscopy so the entire colon can be inspected. It is mandatory to see the rest of the colon because of the chance that there are more polyps farther up in the colon. Then the initial polyp and any others can be removed and a biopsy done at the same time. It is standard practice to remove all polyps at the same time of detection with the colonoscopy, and it would be unethical to leave polyps in place for observation.

The sigmoid colon is the largest part of the large intestine, which is where the majority of polyps and colorectal cancers originate in men. In women, cancer of the colon usually affects the right side of the colon, so screening with sigmoidoscopy may *not* be the most effective test for women.

Endoscopic sigmoidoscopy can be done without a video monitor. The physician peers through the endoscope and searches the inside of the colon. He or she is the only one who sees what is there, and there are often no permanent pictures for you to take with you or for physicians to consult for further study.

Find out if there is video equipment for the procedure or if the doctor will be viewing by eyeball through the endoscopic tube. Most major medical centers and most gastroenterologists will have state-of-the-art equipment with video.

Colonoscopy

Colonoscopy is the most accurate and preferred diagnostic tool for seeing the entire colon up to 95 percent of the time. Many studies have shown that a colonoscopy detects polyps often left undetected by a barium enema X-ray. Also, a physician and a technician perform this procedure simultaneously, so there are two pairs of experienced eyes searching the inside of the colon. Colonoscopy has the highest diagnostic sensitivity and allows a polypectomy—removal of the polyp—to be done at the same time if necessary.

The colonoscope is a fiberoptic tube about the width of your smallest finger and about as long as the colon, up to six feet. Additional instruments can be inserted through this tube, such as a snare of wire loop to sever a polyp with an electrical current. Forceps can be passed through it to remove a piece of tissue from the colon lining for biopsy. A small brush can collect epithelial cells for study under the microscope. A patient could have a small cancer in the cecum, and when it is discovered with colonoscopy and removed right then, the survival rate is high—85 to 90 percent. Colonoscopy is generally an outpatient procedure performed in a doctor's office or an endoscopy suite at a hospital.

Before a Colonoscopy

For a colonoscopy to be effective, the colon must be absolutely clean of fecal matter. This flushing out is done with enemas, with traditional laxatives, or with a nonabsorbable polyethylene glycol (PEG) lavage solution that you drink ahead of time. The oral lavage solution passes through the intestines instead of being absorbed into the urine and causes a liquid stool. There are six or seven different types of oral lavage available and most come in flavors—cherry, lemon-lime, or pineapple—to make them more palatable; but they still taste like salty or soapy water. Your doctor will give you a prescription and tell you which one to buy at your drugstore. Brands commonly prescribed are GoLytely and CoLyte. These lavage solutions come in powdered form in a one-gallon plastic jug that you simply fill with water. You will need to prepare the solution the day before your exam, according to the instructions on the package. Store this in your refrigerator and then have a regular breakfast. Your fasting will begin with lunch, which can be a light liquid, such as soup or broth, and perhaps a gelatin dessert—but it should not be red gelatin because it could mimic the appearance of blood.

Then, between 5:00 P.M. and 6:00 P.M., you will begin drinking the lavage solution, usually an eight-ounce glass every ten to fifteen minutes for about three hours. Prepare to spend the evening near the bathroom because the lavage will flush out your system quickly. It is important to drink an entire glassful every ten or fifteen minutes. If you sip small amounts all during the evening, it will not work as well. Remember, unless your colon is completely cleaned and flushed out, the colonoscopy will not be effective. Poor results could mean you will have to do it again.

If you are at home, you might want to pace yourself with a timer. In the hospital a family member or friend can help you keep track of the intervals. You have three hours to consume all of the lavage. By approximately 9:00 P.M. you should be finished with the last of it, and by 10:00 P.M. you should have emptied your colon, although you might feel bloated or gassy. Get a good night's rest.

Never hesitate to call your doctor if you have any questions or problems with drinking the lavage and getting ready for your colonoscopy. Physicians always expect some phone calls the night before this procedure. Some patients call to ask if they can take the lavage after taking their medications. Some might complain of chills or vomiting, necessitating the physician's attention.

The morning of the colonoscopy, you can have eight ounces of clear liquid such as coffee or tea, clear juice, soup, or water. But don't drink anything within four hours of your exam.

Your physician will need to know about medications you are taking. Aspirin products, arthritis medications, blood thinners, insulin, and iron supplements might be suspended for a period. If you have ever needed antibiotics during dental procedures, let your doctor know. You might need them for a colonoscopy as well to kill any bacteria that might become dislodged during the procedure and invade heart valves, for example.

The Procedure

Before the procedure begins, you might be given an intravenous (IV) narcotic analgesic (painkiller) such as Demerol. An IV sedation such as Valium or Versed might be used to induce a state of "conscious sedation" so you are relaxed. A respiratory monitor, a device called a pulseoximeter, will be clipped on to the end of your finger to measure your pulse and oxygen saturation level during the procedure. Your blood pressure also will be monitored.

Expect your physician to talk with you about any past experience you had with this kind of screening. Your doctor wants you to be comfortable and not apprehensive, and it is reassuring if you have a dialogue with him or her. A caring physician is of utmost importance for the success of this procedure.

Remember, your colon is a tube as long as five feet full of turns and bends, so the trip through it might take from fifteen minutes to an hour. Because you have been sedated, you should not feel any severe discomfort, except for a bit of gas or an urge to move your bowels. The colon, by the way, cannot sense many things that would cause pain, only distension and tugging. You will be lying on your side or your back most of the time while the colonoscope is advancing into your colon, but you might be asked to change position from time to time to move the colonoscope around for better viewing. The colon lining is studied once again while the colonoscope is slowly withdrawn. This procedure is accurate if the patient is well prepared and the physician skilled at moving the colonoscope around.

After the Procedure

Because you have been sedated, you must rest for as long as two hours before you can go home, and somebody must take you home. You will not be allowed to leave on your own, drive a car, or operate machinery. You might feel some abdominal discomfort or distention for several hours after the procedure. Because there is air in your abdominal cavity and diaphragm, you also might have hiccups, feel bloated, or have some cramps caused by the air in your colon. This should disappear quickly with the passage of the gas. Unless a polyp was removed, you should be able to resume normal eating and activity after you leave.

Although colonoscopy is a very invasive examination, complications are rare. Most dreaded is perforation of the colon with the colonoscope, but this is extremely rare. Less serious and more common is hemorrhaging after removal of a polyp or a piece of tissue for biopsy. If you believe something is wrong or if you have a fever or chills, rectal bleeding, or severe abdominal pain after a colonoscopy, call your doctor immediately.

Small-Bowel Enteroscopy

Small-bowel enteroscopy allows direct visualization of the small intestine using an endoscope inserted through the rectum. During the procedure, disorders of the small intestine can be diagnosed and treated, or a biopsy obtained. Intestinal bleeding is the most common reason for this test. It allows the physician to see if bleeding is acute, chronic, or hidden. This test may be especially useful for the evaluation of malabsorption or diarrhea. A sedative and pain medication are normally used for patient comfort.

Capsule Endoscopy or Capsule Camera

Capsule endoscopy, also known as wireless endoscopy or capsule camera, is a new way to see inside the gut. A pill that can be swallowed has its own video camera and light source and will send back images. As the capsule passes through your digestive tract, it sends signals to sensors taped to your abdomen and to a monitor worn on your belt for at least eight hours. This lets your doctor look at the lining of the small intestine—duodenum, jejunum, ileum—the parts that cannot be reached by upper endoscopy or colonoscopy. For the first time, doctors are able to see parts of the digestive tract that previously could only be seen at surgery or autopsy. One thing it revealed is that the incidence of damage in the small bowel induced by nonsteroidal anti-inflammatory drugs (NSAIDs) is much higher than previously thought. This came from a study of forty arthritis patients who took NSAIDs daily for at least three months prior to the study.

Capsule endoscopy usually is done to search for a cause of bleeding from the small intestine, or for polyps, inflammatory bowel disease, Crohn's disease, ulcers, or tumors of the small intestine. The test requires fasting for twelve hours. Complications are rare, but a potential risk is obstruction of the capsule. Signs of this would include bloating, pain, or vomiting.

The downside of capsule endoscopy is that the capsule continues on its passage and cannot be stopped temporarily to take a second look at a particular site, or to take a tissue sample for biopsy.

Because this is a new diagnostic procedure, not all insurance companies cover it yet.

Endoscopic Ultrasonography

Endoscopic ultrasonography (EUS) is even more precise than external ultrasound. An echoendoscope can be inserted into your digestive tract to send sound waves and images back directly from the site. It provides more detailed pictures of the anatomy of the digestive tract. The echoendoscope is also good at finding small stones in the gallbladder and common bile duct that cannot be detected by conventional ultrasound. It can be used to diagnose the cause of abdominal pain or weight loss. It also is used to evaluate an abnormality such as a growth that was detected at a prior endoscopy or X-ray. The extent of cancers of the digestive tract and respiratory system also can be seen.

Endoscopic ultrasound is increasingly employed and may be used to guide fine-needle biopsy. Abnormal-appearing lymph nodes and tumors lying beneath the lining of the esophagus, stomach, and intestine can be biopsied in this way.

Depending on the area of interest, the tube is inserted either through the mouth or through the anus. The ultrasound probe can be placed next to a rectal, esophageal, stomach, or pancreatic tumor, and the size and depth of the tumor can be determined. This tumor staging is important in treatment decisions.

As with most endoscopic tests, this one requires fasting overnight before the procedure.

Diagnostic Endoscopy and Health Insurance: Why You Need to Be Well Informed

Even if the gastroenterologist you choose is included in your health insurance plan, some of the affiliated services, such as endoscopic testing or biopsy, may not be covered. The type of treatment often depends on the type of insurance. For example, depending upon your insurance, you may have to get a colonoscopy with injections of local painkillers, rather than with more sophisticated anesthesia. Most people are not aware of this.

Medical insurance usually covers the cost of biopsy procedures, laboratory tests, and pathology fees, but not always all of them. Health maintenance organizations (HMOs) often require that biopsies be done only by certain laboratories with whom they have contracts, and the place your physician has chosen to have your pathology study done might not be one of them.

Tests will cost several hundred dollars, so check to be sure that the particular pathology lab accepts your medical insurance. If not, discuss this with your doctor and find out what other alternatives you have. You might be able to negotiate a reduced charge if your surgeon prefers to use that particular lab. It is not uncommon for your surgeon to be part of your medical plan coverage, but not the laboratory, even if they operate in the same medical center.

Suppose you have an endoscopic examination in your doctor's office, and a polyp is removed, but the hospital's pathology fee is not covered by your insurance. Your insurer will only pay for pathology done by an outside commercial lab. However, if you are in a comprehensive cancer center, your surgeon will not be able to make a surgical decision based on an outside commercial laboratory biopsy. He or she will want one done in the same place where the screening was done. Outside commercial labs are often acceptable to doctors for analysis of potassium levels and other blood tests but not for anything as critical as a tissue biopsy. If your biopsy was done at an outside commercial lab, your surgeon must get the biopsy slides from another lab or hospital and then have them analyzed again by his or her hospital pathology staff. This will double the cost of the biopsy, and the insurance will likely not cover it.

Doctors are used to working with other doctors they know as a part of a multidisciplinary team to treat a patient. Mutual trust, a common hospital, complementary training, and professional competence are part of the "glue" holding together these teams. Current trends in health insurance do not necessarily recognize these groups, and the teams might be fragmented if one or more doctors necessary to your care are not covered in your plan. This sometimes results in excess strain on the doctor-patient relationship if access to what is perceived as necessary or desirable by health-care providers is limited by health insurance coverage.

If you or your doctor want a second pathology opinion   Just as the choice of pathology laboratory could be limited by your health insurance coverage, your choice of pathologist also could be limited by your physician. The pathologist and lab that provide the study and the report on your case are usually chosen by your gastroenterologist and surgeon or hospital. Rarely are you asked if you would like to choose your own pathologist or lab.

Pathology labs have been known to make mistakes, so talk it over with your doctor if you want to double-check results. It is not uncommon for patients with carcinoma involving a polyp to want another opinion, especially if the biopsy shows that cancer has not broken into the colon wall, but there were cancer cells in the stalk of the polyp. Ask your gastroenterologist to help you arrange for your slides to be reviewed by different pathologists to obtain second and often third opinions on what to do next.

Your tissue samples are kept on glass slides and in paraffin blocks in the lab's pathology department. They are part of your medical records, and you can have them sent to another pathologist. Hospital labs keep these tissue samples for many years. You will probably have to give the lab twenty-four hours' notice in writing or sign a hospital form so they can release the slides and a written report.

Always be sure to find out ahead of time just what complications you are likely to run into. You will want to know that you are getting the best possible treatment—indeed, the proper treatment.

PART II

Medical Treatment for Disorders and Diseases of the Gastrointestinal System

Chapter 4
The Esophagus

THE ESOPHAGUS, sometimes known as the gullet, doesn't really do anything exotic. It's a hollow muscular tube through which food is transported from your mouth to your stomach, with the help of automatic muscular contractions known as peristalsis. Nevertheless, it can develop problems that you'll learn about in this section:

- Gastroesophageal reflux disease
- Esophagitis and infections
- Barrett's esophagus
- Mechanical disorders: hiatal hernia, strictures, and diverticula
- Motility disorders: spasm and achalasia
- Food impaction and perforation
- Scleroderma
- Benign tumors and cancer

Gastroesophageal Reflux Disease

Almost everybody experiences heartburn once in a while, but as many as fifteen million Americans have discovered that what they thought was heartburn or indigestion is actually more serious. It's a condition called gastroesophageal reflux disease (GERD)—more commonly known as reflux disease. *Gastro* refers to the stomach, and *reflux* means to flow back, so gastroesophageal reflux is the return of the stomach's contents back up into the esophagus. If your body fails to prevent this acidic mixture from backing up into the esophagus, the lining of your esophagus can be damaged. Stomach acid is more potent than battery acid, and the esophagus is not prepared to handle it.

Reflux disease is increasing dramatically, yet many people wait years to get proper diagnosis and take steps to cure it. While the cause in some cases is yet unknown, others can be directly linked to lifestyle—obesity, increased consumption of fatty foods, lack of exercise, and smoking. However, reflux disease also can be caused by a congenital defect in the esophageal valve, trauma, a medical condition, or certain medications.

According to the National Institutes of Health, more than sixty million adults experience reflux disease and heartburn at least once a month, and about twenty-five million adults suffer daily from heartburn. Twenty-five percent of pregnant women experience daily heartburn, and more than 50 percent have occasional distress. Recent studies show that reflux disease in infants and children is more common than previously recognized and may produce recurrent vomiting, coughing, and other respiratory problems, or failure to thrive.

The lower esophageal sphincter (LES) is a high-pressure muscular zone serving as a valve at the bottom of the esophagus. In normal digestion, it opens—to the size of a quarter or wider—to allow food to pass into the stomach. It then closes to prevent food and acidic stomach juices from flowing back into the esophagus. Reflux disease occurs when the LES is weak or relaxes inappropriately and allows the stomach's contents to flow up into the esophagus. The severity of reflux disease depends on the severity of the LES dysfunction, the normal peristaltic activity to cleanse the bottom of the esophagus, as well as on the type and amount of fluid brought up from the stomach and the neutralizing effect of saliva. Saliva contains water, electrolytes, enzymes, and mucus, which neutralize and coat swallowed food to ease its passage through the esophagus. LES muscular tone may be reduced by medications that dilate blood vessels, such as nitrates and calcium channel blockers used to control high blood pressure. Smoking also affects it in a negative way.

Risk Factors for Reflux Disease

Reflux disease can happen at any age but more commonly happens in middle age or later. It's been suggested that the rising incidence of this disease coincides with higher rates of obesity and with people eating fattier foods. Here are some risk factors.

Smoking is implicated in nearly every health condition known to modern society. It is a primary risk factor in reflux disease because it works to weaken the muscle of the LES.

Alcohol abuse also can be blamed. It does the same thing as smoking—weakens the LES. And if you smoke and drink in excess, you make the risk much worse. The sum of these two addictions is apparently greater than their parts.

Certain medications such as nitrates, Fosamax, and calcium channel blockers can weaken the sphincter muscles. If you've been taking calcium channel blockers to treat your high blood pressure for several years, you also may experience reflux disease. Other drugs that put you at risk for reflux disease include nitroglycerin for angina; theophylline for asthma; B-receptor agonists; anticholinergics; and benzodiazepines, which are sedatives and antianxiety drugs. Be especially cognizant of reflux symptoms.

Hiatal hernia occurs when the upper part of the stomach moves up into the chest through a small opening in the diaphragm, the muscle that separates your stomach from your chest. This opening in the diaphragm muscle is known as the hiatus. New studies show that the opening in the diaphragm acts as an additional sphincter around the lower end of the esophagus. Many otherwise healthy people age fifty and older have a small hiatal hernia, simply from the wear and tear of life. However, hiatal hernias affect people of all ages. Pregnant women may get them because of the added weight and pressure from nearby organs. Coughing, vomiting, straining, or sudden physical exertion can cause increased pressure in the abdomen and result in hiatal hernia. These hernias usually don't require treatment unless there is danger of becoming strangulated (twisted in a way that cuts off blood supply) or they are complicated by severe reflux disease or esophagitis. In such cases, surgery can reduce the size of the hernia to prevent strangulation. (See chapter 11 for more about hiatal hernia.)

Obesity is a risk factor. The more fat cells there are clogging up your middle, the more difficult it is for your digestive organs to work properly. Compare it with being squished in an overcrowded elevator or subway car at rush hour.

Eradication of Helicobacter pylori. For reasons we don't fully understand, the bacterium that is responsible for ulcers and gastritis, *H. pylori*, also may guard us against reflux disease. So naturally, if you kill it off by treating ulcers, you may put yourself at risk for reflux disease.

Other risks include esophageal dysmotility, or problems with the automatic muscle contractions of the esophagus (see page 69) and hyperacidity in the stomach.

Symptoms of Reflux Disease

Heartburn and queasy stomach are two of the most common symptoms of reflux disease. Heartburn usually feels like a burning chest pain beginning behind the breastbone and moving upward to the neck and throat. It feels as if food is coming back into your mouth, leaving an acid or bitter taste. The burning, pressure, or pain of heartburn can last as long as two hours and usually is worse after eating. Hunger pains also may be a symptom of reflux disease, as is upper digestive gas and bloating, or a feeling of fullness.

Other symptoms include:

- Unexplained chest pain, often at night. Sometimes heartburn can be mistaken for the pain of heart disease or a heart attack, but there are differences. Exercise may aggravate pain from heart disease, and rest may relieve the pain. Pain from heartburn is less closely associated with physical activity.

- Increased symptoms when lying down and when eating. Reflux when bending over may be caused by a mechanical failure of the sphincter muscle. Many people get relief by standing upright or taking an antacid, which clears acid out of the esophagus.

- Difficulty swallowing (dysphagia).

- Reflux-induced asthma may be caused by aspiration of gastric contents to the lung, leading to bronchospasm. It is critical to distinguish asthma from reflux disease, as it will influence treatment decisions.

- Chronic cough and hoarseness.

- Tooth erosion has been attributed to acid reflux by some.

- Vomiting blood or passing blood in stool (this is an emergency).

Complications from Reflux Disease

Over time, reflux disease, left untreated, can lead to complications such as an ulcer or stricture of the esophagus, erosive esophagitis, or Barrett's esophagus.

Esophagitis

A third of people with reflux disease have esophagitis. Of this number, 40 percent will resolve spontaneously, 50 percent have chronic disease, and 10 percent will progress to Barrett's esophagus—a precancerous condition where the delicate lining of the esophagus takes on the appearance and characteristics of the tough lining of the stomach.

When stomach acid and digestive enzymes repeatedly reflux into the esophagus, the lining becomes inflamed. This inflammation is known as esophagitis and can cause bleeding, which shows up in anemia, black stools, and vomiting blood. When it is severe, esophageal ulcers develop, and swallowing may cause pain when food touches that area of the esophagus. When it goes on for a long time, esophagitis can result in scarring and narrowing of the esophagus.

Radiation treatment for breast cancer, as well as swallowing caustic substances such as lye, also can cause esophagitis. Other causes include cigarette smoking, obesity, alcohol, and certain medications such as non-steroidal anti-inflammatory drugs (NSAIDs), calcium channel blockers, and beta-blockers.

The usual endoscopic tests can find esophagitis, but it is important to get a biopsy of the inflamed tissue because cancer of the esophagus can mimic this condition. Also, a biopsy will reveal any precancerous changes.

Pill Esophagitis

People who take many medications can develop pill esophagitis. It is caused by frequent contact of medication with the delicate esophageal lining. This often is seen in nursing homes, where elderly residents often take multiple medications. Fosamax, antibiotics, potassium chloride, NSAIDs, quinidine, and emperonium bromide account for 90 percent of reported cases. It also can occur after chemotherapy. Treatment is the same as for reflux disease and people are advised to drink lots of water with their medications.

Stricture

The LES opens to the size of a quarter or wider. However, recurrent inflammation and scarring may make the underlying tissues fibrous, and the opening narrows. This narrowing, or stricture, can be severe in advanced cases. In fact, the opening may shrink to the size of a very thin pencil. Food and fluid only move slowly across the opening into the stomach. Think of a clogged sink drain. A large piece of food, such as meat, may completely block the esophagus (see page 76). Correct diagnosis is important, since cancer also can narrow the esophagus in the same way.

Barrett's Esophagus

Barrett's esophagus can develop if you've had reflux disease or esophagitis for many years. This condition represents cellular change in the lining of the esophagus and is a precursor to esophageal cancer. Cells that line the esophagus are called squamous cells. With Barrett's esophagus, these cells turn into specialized columnar cells, not usually found in this location. Once the cells change—a process called metaplasia—they will very rarely revert to normal. These abnormal changes damage the lining of the esophagus, which sometimes becomes thick and hardened. This causes strictures, or narrowing, that can prevent food and liquid from reaching the stomach. So far, there is no cure for this disease, so the goal of treatment is to prevent further damage by stopping any acid reflux from the stomach.

The molecular changes in this condition are now being investigated. For example, mutations in the p53 gene show an overexpression of certain cells—a continuation of progression from esophagitis to metaplasia to dysplasia to neoplasia. Dysplasia is the alteration in size, shape, and organization of cells. And neoplasia is abnormal new growth—or cancer.

Who Is at Risk?   Men over forty-five are at the highest risk for Barrett's esophagus, although others also can get it. If you've had reflux disease for five to ten years, your risk is high. Having severe esophagitis in a large area of the esophagus—say, greater than eight centimeters (three inches)—puts you at increased risk. Also, if you have an ulceration or stricture of the esophagus, you may be predisposed to Barrett's esophagus.

Will It Lead to Cancer?   About 5 to 10 percent of people with Barrett's develop esophageal cancer, and because of this risk, you need to have endoscopic screening regularly to watch for any changes in the esophageal tissue. Recent data suggest that chronic esophagitis is needed to progress to Barrett's esophagus, and from there the displastic areas are considered premalignant or frankly malignant. Current theories hold that treatment with proton pump inhibitors or surgery may reduce the risk of progression of the disease.

Getting a Diagnosis

Once you and your doctor have determined the presence of symptoms and risk factors, you may be put on antireflux and/or antiacid medication. A clinical trial found that if using this therapy for two to three weeks reduced or eliminated symptoms, the patient most likely had reflux disease. This is a good way to determine whether you need further tests. However, if this does not help, further tests are indicated.

- *A pH probe worn in the esophagus* is the gold standard diagnostic test for reflux disease. By monitoring you for twenty-four-hour periods, your doctor can determine if the acidity level of your esophagus and your symptoms change during meals, activity, and sleep. The probe is attached to a recording device worn outside the body.

- *Esophageal manometry* will test the muscle tone and peristalsis of your esophagus. This helps identify critically low pressure in the LES or abnormalities in muscle contraction. This entails swallowing a catheter for about one hour. Pressure changes are recorded on graph paper.

- *Upper endoscopy* will locate abnormalities in the mucous membrane, cellular changes, Barrett's metaplasia, or any other complications. By placing a small lighted tube with a tiny video camera at the end into the esophagus, the doctor may see inflammation or irritation of the tissue lining the esophagus (esophagitis). If the findings are abnormal or questionable, biopsy can be done by removing a piece of tissue. This test should be considered if you have ongoing and/or controlled reflux symptoms, particularly if you are over fifty. (See chapter 3 for more detail on this test.)

Treating Reflux Disease

Therapy without drugs is generally not effective. Although most people need to change their lifestyle for long-term relief from reflux disease, that won't be effective immediately, especially if there is already damage to the esophageal tissue or LES. You need a jump start with a program of medications that provide immediate relief so the condition doesn't get worse.

Antacids such as TUMS or Maalox are okay for occasional indigestion to provide temporary or partial relief by neutralizing acid in the esophagus. However, long-term use of antacids can result in side effects such as diarrhea, altered calcium metabolism, and a buildup of magnesium and aluminum in the body. Too much magnesium and aluminum can be serious for people with kidney disease. Today there are more effective medications both over the counter and by prescription.

Acid Suppression Therapy

First try H-2 blockers. These medications block histamine, a natural chemical in your body that stimulates stomach acid secretion. They prevent the histamine from attaching to your stomach cells that make acid. H-2 blockers are available without prescription and provide symptomatic relief in more than 60 percent of people; about 30 percent are healed by them. Initially these drugs should be used in high doses twice a day for four weeks. Then they can be decreased to once a day for the next six to eight weeks.

Over-the-counter H-2 blockers include:

- Pepcid AC
- Tagamet HB
- Zantac 75
- Axid AR

Side effects from these medications are minimal, but people with worrisome symptoms such as weight loss, nausea, vomiting, bleeding, and dysphagia should consult their physicians, as should pregnant women.

Proton Pump Inhibitors

Proton pump inhibitors (PPIs) attack the problem another way. They block the production of stomach acid altogether by shutting down a system in the stomach known as the proton pump. These drugs are the mainstay of therapy for reflux disease and are very safe if you have moderate to severe symptoms. They also are effective in complicated esophagitis, Barrett's esophagus, or esophageal ulceration or stricture. PPIs are more effective than H-2 blockers, and more than 90 percent of those who take them find relief and healing. In combination with other drugs, they also are used to treat the *H. pylori* infection of stomach ulcers (see page 88). They include:

- Prilosec
- Prevacid
- AcipHex
- Protonix
- Nexium
- Rapinex

PPIs, available only by prescription, come in capsules, tablets, and powder. One of them also can be injected intravenously in the hospital. Most people take these drugs for a month or two, but some may need to take them longer. Long-term treatment is safe and effective for refractory reflux esophagitis. PPIs are as effective as surgical therapy for complicated reflux disease and for symptoms.

Once you stop taking them, your symptoms may come back, however. Arthur is fifty and has long-standing symptoms of heartburn. He is otherwise in good health and there are no "worry" symptoms, such as difficulty or pain swallowing, weight loss, or vomiting. After a thorough checkup, he was put on a four-week trial of oral PPI and some lifestyle modifications. Whenever he stops taking the medications, however, the symptoms return. An endoscopy revealed a mild redness in the lower end of his esophagus, but a biopsy showed no *H. pylori* or precancerous cells. He remained on the medication for eight months and is symptom-free. He wants to know if it is safe to continue on this medication.

If You Take Other Medications

Be careful of interactions with PPIs. Don't use any other drugs, including over-the-counter herbal remedies, before talking with your doctor. If you take medications for epilepsy or prevention of blood clots, the effect of these drugs may be increased when you also take a proton pump inhibitor. Antifungal drugs to treat nail bed fungus infections may not be absorbed as well if you are using PPIs. The breakdown of Valium may be blocked by some of the PPIs.

Monitoring PPI Use

If you must take PPIs for more than six months, then you and your doctor may want you to have periodic blood tests to monitor your gastrin and vitamin B_{12} levels. You also may need an upper endoscopy every two years to monitor for damage to the esophageal lining.

Vitamin B_{12} Supplements

Long-term acid suppression reduces your ability to absorb vitamin B_{12} from your food, so your doctor may advise you to take supplements. This vitamin maintains healthy nerve cells and red blood cells and also is used to make our DNA, the genetic material in our cells. It also is important in the metabolism of fats, protein and carbohydrates. Most of us get enough vitamin B_{12} in our daily diet in animal foods such as milk, fish, meat, and eggs, or in fortified breakfast cereals. Vitamin B_{12} binds to the protein in our food. Normally, stomach acid releases B_{12} from protein during digestion. Once released, the B_{12} combines with a substance called the intrinsic factor before it is absorbed in the bloodstream. If you are taking medications that stop your stomach from producing the acid, then this natural system is disturbed.

Without enough B_{12} in your diet, you may feel weak and tired, nauseated, constipated, or gassy. A deficiency can cause you to lose your appetite and lose weight and can cause neurological changes such as numbness and tingling in your hands and feet. Depression, confusion, difficulty with balance, memory loss, and a sore mouth or tongue also indicate vitamin B_{12} deficiency.

It takes quite a while to deplete the body's supply of this vitamin, so talk with your doctor about the long-term picture. If you cannot get enough in your food, vitamin B_{12} supplements or injections may be necessary.

Side Effects

Proton pump inhibitors generally don't cause problems, but side effects include diarrhea, constipation, gas, abdominal pain, nausea, and headaches. In rare cases PPIs may cause allergic reactions such as itching, dizziness, muscle pain, or blurred vision. In some people long-term use can lead to gastrointestinal infections because stomach acid helps kill bacteria in the stomach—and the PPI stops acid production. If you notice tarry stools or you vomit blood or a substance that resembles coffee grounds, call your doctor right away. These are signs of intestinal bleeding.

Who Should Not Take PPIs?

If you have liver or kidney problems, or if you are pregnant or breast-feeding, your doctor may want to limit your use of PPIs.

Laparoscopic Surgery

Laparoscopic surgical treatment to strengthen the LES is rarely indicated for reflux disease. However, it is sometimes considered for very young patients with severe reflux or for those who cannot tolerate the medications due to side effects or allergies. Surgery should not be considered until all other measures have been tried. According to a five-year clinical study reported in the *Journal of the American College of Surgery* in 2001, 25 to 50 percent of surgical patients may still have to take PPIs or antacids to control symptoms of reflux disease.

Janet, a fifty-five-year-old housewife with Barrett's esophagus (without dysplasia) and severe symptoms of heartburn, had tried all available PPIs for nearly a year. Although they alleviated her symptoms, she was experiencing headaches and diarrhea with each of the PPIs. This has naturally discouraged her from continuing, and she and her doctor are considering laparoscopic surgery.

Laparoscopic Fundoplication

This is a safe procedure in which part of the stomach is wrapped around the back of the esophagus to create a one-way valve in the esophagus to allow food to pass into the stomach but to prevent stomach acid from flowing into the esophagus.

The EndoCinch Suturing System

This creates pleats at the LES. It's like a tiny sewing machine attached to the end of a flexible endoscope and allows the doctor to stitch near the LES. Two stitches can be placed and tied together to create a pleat. Other suturing techniques include the full-thickness placation system, and the Sew-Right device.

The Stretta Catheter

This is a disposable, flexible catheter with needle electrodes that delivers precise radio-frequency energy to the LES. It is inserted through the mouth and advanced to the junction of the esophagus and the stomach. A balloon is inflated, and needle electrodes are deployed into the tissue. The radio-frequency energy creates thermal lesions in the muscle of the LES. As these lesions heal, the tissue contracts and reduces reflux episodes.

Endoscopic Implants

The Enteryx technique and the Gatekeeper technique both involve implanting substances into the esophagus that help block the reflux of stomach acids. The Enteryx is made of polymer and a solvent permanently implanted into the wall of the lower esophagus. By strengthening the muscle that separates the lower part of the esophagus from the stomach, it forms a barrier. Using an endoscope, the liquid polymer is injected into the muscle of the LES with a needle catheter. The polymer will solidify into a spongelike permanent implant.

The Gatekeeper technique is used in Europe and was expected to be approved for use in the United States soon. This is a prosthesis made of material similar to that used for contact lenses. With an endoscope it is placed into the esophageal wall while it is dry. Once it contacts moisture, it expands and forms a barrier that helps keep food in the stomach.

Treating a Stricture

To treat esophageal stricture, the lumen, or hollow space, is gently but forcefully opened or dilated. Dilation is often performed in conjunction with an upper endoscopy exam. Here are some ways it can be done:

- *Bougie:* A series of increasingly larger, soft rubber or plastic weighted dilators are moved across the stricture, gently opening it.

- *Guide wire:* A thin wire, placed across the stricture, is used to guide increasingly wider dilators over it.

- *Balloons:* Different types of sausage-shaped balloons can be placed across the stricture. The balloon is forcefully inflated to open the narrowed area.

Your doctor will choose the most appropriate method for you. The only alternative to dilation is surgery. Dilation always causes minimal bleeding, although it is rarely excessive. A rare but serious complication would be perforation or tearing of the esophagus. This would require surgery to correct.

John, seventy, had a long-standing history of GERD, but recently experienced difficulty with solid food sticking in his gullet. A video-esophagram was done to observe the swallowing process and esophageal function, an upper endoscopy with biopsy, and a CT scan of his chest to discover a peptic stricture in the distal esophagus. There was no evidence of cancer, so John had a bougie dilation of the stricture just days prior to embarking on a cruise to Alaska with his wife for their fiftieth anniversary.

Treating Barrett's Esophagus

If acid suppression medications like H-2 agonists and PPIs don't work to control Barrett's esophagus, then other therapy is called for. With low-grade dysplasia—the alteration in the size, shape, and organization of cells—monitoring and taking a biopsy every year or two may be all that is required. This means we can see cell alteration at or near its beginning. High-grade dysplasia can be treated by surgically removing the affected area and monitoring it closely with endoscopy. Managing high-grade dysplasia is controversial. Treatment options include removing the esophagus, or experimental therapies such as ablation therapy. Not everyone who has high-grade dysplasia will develop cancer when they are monitored for years with endoscopic biopsies. This makes the treatment choice difficult.

- *Esophagectomy*, removal of the esophagus, is successful in curing esophageal cancer. Proponents for surgery argue that people with Barrett's esophagus will avoid cancer in this way. But a significant number of these patients may not get cancer. Although some small cancers may be missed by such surveillance, most are not.

- *Photodynamic therapy (PDT)* involves administering a light-sensitive drug (photosensitizer) through the patient's vein or by mouth. This makes all the cells in the body hypersensitive to light exposure, including the Barrett's esophagus cells. Then a laser is used to destroy those cells. This treatment makes the Barrett's cells die and fall off the esophagus wall. Follow-up medication is used to control reflux and allow the normal esophageal lining to grow back.

- *Thermal ablation*, like PDT, destroys the Barrett's cells. This therapy uses heat via electrical probe, lasers, or a gas to directly burn the Barrett's lining off.

- *Endoscopic mucosal resection* is an experimental therapy used mostly to treat cancer, but it also can be used to treat high-grade dysplasia if it involves only a small area of esophageal lining. This is done through an endoscope; the procedure lifts the Barrett's lining by injecting a solution under it or applying suction, much like a colon polyp removal.

Leonard is fifty-two and had been taking over-the-counter antacids for what he thought was heartburn for more than ten years. When he finally went to the doctor, he was put on PPIs and showed immediate improvement. He was also referred to a gastroenterologist for an upper endoscopy. This test revealed that Leonard had Barrett's esophagus with a high-grade neoplasia or cancer in situ, meaning it had not spread beyond the esophagus. He underwent esophageal surgery and after two years of follow-up is doing fine.

Lifestyle Changes and Prevention

Although the medications will reduce the amount of reflux and reduce damage to the esophageal lining, you face an uphill battle unless you reduce risk factors that you can control, such as smoking, overeating, or late-night snacking. There are many ways you can avoid weakening the LES and irritating any inflammation in your esophagus.

- Cigarette smoking weakens the LES, so quitting is important in reducing symptoms.
- Find substitutes for medications that relax the LES, such as nitrates, calcium channel blockers, and anticholinergic agents.
- Avoid food and beverages that can weaken the LES, such as chocolate, peppermint, fatty foods, coffee, and alcoholic beverages.
- Avoid foods and beverages that can irritate a damaged esophageal lining, such as citrus fruits and juices, tomato products, and pepper.

- Reduce portion sizes at mealtime.
- Stand up and walk around after eating.
- Don't eat late at night. Eat meals at least two to three hours before bedtime to lessen reflux by allowing the acid in the stomach to decrease and your stomach to empty partially.
- Maintain a healthy weight. Being overweight often worsens symptoms of reflux disease.
- Elevate the head of your bed, not just by leaning on more pillows but also by raising the bed itself at the head on six-inch blocks. If this is impossible, look for a specially designed wedge to put under your mattress. This elevation reduces heartburn by allowing gravity to minimize reflux of stomach contents.
- Eliminate excessive bending, lifting, and abdominal exercises.
- Don't crowd your middle with girdles and tight belts, all of which increase abdominal pressure and provoke reflux.

Benign Esophageal Tumors and Cancer

The esophagus can sprout a large number and variety of benign tumors, but the vast majority are extremely rare and usually don't produce clinical disease. They grow from the lining of the esophagus or from the muscular wall.

Leiomyoma is the most common benign esophageal tumor. It may cause difficulty in swallowing and chest pain, but in most cases there are no symptoms and it rarely bleeds, as this tumor does if in the stomach. It can be seen with a barium X-ray as a smooth, round defect projecting from one wall of the esophagus. These tumors need to be removed only if they cause trouble such as difficulty or pain with swallowing.

Squamous cell papillomas have frondlike projections and develop at several sites in the esophagus simultaneously. They rarely grow large enough to produce problems with swallowing. Except when associated with tylosis, a hardening of the skin, these lesions are not considered precancerous.

Fibrovascular polyps consist of a core of loose, fibrous connective tissue, fat, and blood vessels covered by a thick layer of squamous epithelium (the cells that line the esophagus). Such a polyp may become quite large, with a very long stalk that permits it to flop back and forth in the esophagus. People have actually regurgitated the free end of the polyp into the mouth. In some cases, the regurgitated polyp has caused sudden death by obstructing the larynx.

Granular cell tumors grow under the lining of the esophagus and usually don't protrude. Usually they are discovered incidentally during endoscopy and rarely cause symptoms, although there have been occasional reports of difficult swallowing because of large tumors. In that case, they would have to be removed. There also have been rare reports of malignant granular cell tumors in the esophagus.

Esophageal Cancer

The most common esophageal tumor, however, is the squamous cell carcinoma, a cancer that has one of the lowest survival rates. This type typically appears in a black man sixty to seventy years old with a history of alcoholism and/or smoking. Usually it's found in the upper half of the esophagus.

The other common cancer is adenocarcinoma, which is common in both white and black men fifty to sixty years old. Usually this is due to Barrett's metaplasia progressing from reflux disease and is found in the lower half of the esophagus. All other cancers of the esophagus are rare. It has been increasing alarmingly in industrialized nations in recent decades compared to other squamous cell cancers and all other cancers. We're not sure why, but the increase may be linked to the redistribution of *H. pylori*, the bacterium that is responsible for stomach ulcers. By successfully treating ulcers we kill the *H. pylori*, which may have protected us from reflux disease and thus its complications. Medical scientists also believe that smoking and the obesity epidemic are contributing factors to the rising incidence of esophageal adenocarcinoma.

Generally there are no symptoms early in the disease, but as esophageal cancer develops, symptoms similar to reflux disease develop such as reflux, regurgitation, and difficult or painful swallowing. Other symptoms include severe weight loss; pain in the throat or back, behind the breastbone, or between the shoulder blades; hoarseness or chronic cough; vomiting; and coughing up blood.

If the cancer spreads outside the esophagus, it first goes to the lymph nodes—small, bean-shaped structures that are part of your body's immune system. Esophageal cancer, however, can spread to almost any other part of the body, including the liver, lungs, brain, and bones.

Risk Factors for Esophageal Cancer

Many people who have the risk factors never get esophageal cancer, and sometimes those who do get it, have none of the known risks. Given that, there are still risks we can pinpoint.

Age and sex are both risk factors. Like many cancers, esophageal cancer is more likely to occur as you get older. Most people who develop esophageal cancer are over sixty, and it is more common in men than in women. Cigarette smoking and heavy use of alcohol are risk factors, and if you smoke and drink heavily, your risk is especially high. It's believed that these substances increase each other's harmful effects. Less common risks include swallowing lye or other caustic substances that damage the esophagus. If you've had head or neck cancers, you are at increased risk.

There are some risks that can be quantified. For example, if you have achalasia, a rare motility disorder of the esophagus (see page 69), your risk of esophageal cancer increases 16 times. Here are some of the numbers:

If you have	*Your risk is increased*
Achalasia	16 times
Reflux disease (depending on length of time)	up to 7 times
Radiation therapy for breast cancer	up to 5 times
Increased body mass index or obesity	up to 4.3 times
Hiatal hernia	4 times
Esophageal ulcer or esophagitis	4 times
Long-term use of drugs that weaken the LES*	3.8 times
Difficulty swallowing (dysphagia)	2 times
More than four prescriptions for H-2 blockers	1.5 times
H. pylori	controversial

*These include nitroglycerin for heart disease; theophylline and B-receptor agonists for asthma; anticholinergics; and benzodiazepines.

Diagnosing Esophageal Cancer

Because the symptoms can be mistaken for heartburn or reflux disease, esophageal cancer often has progressed and metastasized before it is diagnosed. Once cancer is revealed, more tests are needed to determine if the cancer has spread and to determine its stage.

Barium swallow (videoesophagram)   This is a series of X-rays of the esophagus. After drinking a liquid containing barium that coats the inside of the esophagus, X-rays show any changes in the shape of the esophagus.

Endoscopy with biopsy   If an abnormal area is found, the doctor can collect cells and tissue through the endoscope for examination under a microscope. A biopsy can ascertain cancer or tissue changes that may lead to cancer, as well as other conditions.

CT scan (computed tomography) Once cancer is found, a CT scan is done to check for metastasis. A computer linked to an X-ray machine creates a series of detailed pictures of areas inside the body. (These tests are described in chapter 3.)

Bone scan   This also tracks the spread of cancer. Images of bones on a computer screen or on film show whether the cancer has spread to the bones. A small amount of radioactive substance is injected into a vein; it travels through the bloodstream and collects in the bones, especially in areas of abnormal bone growth. An instrument called a scanner measures the radioactivity levels in these areas.

Bronchoscopy   By inserting a thin tube—bronchoscope—into your nose or mouth, the doctor can look down into your windpipe and other breathing passages to check for the presence of cancer.

Staging Esophageal Cancer

If cancer is discovered, the doctor needs to know the extent of the disease. This is called staging. It is a careful attempt to find out whether the cancer has spread and, if so, to what parts of the body. Knowing the stage of the disease helps plan treatment, which depends on the size of the tumor as well as how aggressive it is, and whether cancer has spread.

> *Stage I.*   The cancer is only in the top layers of cells lining the esophagus.

> *Stage II.*   The cancer involves deeper layers of the lining of the esophagus, or it has spread to nearby lymph nodes. The cancer has not spread to other parts of the body.

> *Stage III.*   The cancer has invaded more deeply into the wall of the esophagus or has spread to tissues or lymph nodes near the esophagus. It has not spread to other parts of the body.

Stage IV. The cancer has spread to other parts of the body. Esophageal cancer can spread almost anywhere in the body, including the liver, lungs, brain, and bones.

Treating Esophageal Cancer

The mainstay of treatment for esophageal cancer is to surgically remove the tumor. Sometimes the entire esophagus is removed. Chemotherapy, radiation, photodynamic therapy, and combination therapies are performed. The type of treatment depends on the extent of the tumor and your general health. In a comprehensive cancer center you would be treated by a team of specialists, who may include a gastroenterologist, surgeon, medical oncologist, and radiation oncologist. Many different treatments or combinations of treatment may be used to control the cancer and/or to improve quality of life by reducing symptoms. Here's what the latest studies show.

- Combined surgery, chemotherapy, and radiation are superior to surgery alone. One-year survival rates were sixteen months for multimodal therapy versus eleven months for surgery. The three-year survival was 32 percent, versus 6 percent for surgery alone.

- Chemotherapy drugs Cisplatin and 5-FU added to radiation are better than radiation alone for people with Stage III disease. The five-year survival rate was 26 percent compared to 0 percent for radiation alone.

- The three-year survival rate was 40 percent for both multimodal and surgery alone in people with Stage I or II disease. Disease-free survival was slightly better for multimodal group than surgery alone.

Before Surgery

Because cancer treatment may make the mouth sensitive and at risk for infection, doctors often advise patients with esophageal cancer to see a dentist for a dental exam and treatment before cancer treatment begins. Preparation for this surgery includes an endoscopic examination; bone scan; pulmonary function tests; CT scan of the chest, abdomen, and pelvis; and others.

Surgery

This is the most common treatment for esophageal cancer. Usually the surgeon removes the tumor along with all or part of the esophagus and any nearby lymph nodes. Removing the entire esophagus is called esophagectomy. If only part of the esophagus is removed, the remaining healthy part is connected to the stomach so you can swallow. Sometimes a part of the intestine is used to make the connection. The surgeon also may widen the opening between the stomach and the small intestine to allow stomach contents to pass more easily into the small intestine. Sometimes surgery is performed after other treatment is finished.

Surgery may cause short-term pain and tenderness in the area, but this discomfort is controlled with medication. You may be taught special breathing and coughing exercises to keep your lungs clear. This involves techniques taught by a clinical physical therapist.

Chemotherapy

Sometimes chemotherapy is used before surgery or other treatment to try to reduce the size of the tumor. These drugs usually are given by IV injection. When used after surgery or other treatment, it is called adjuvant chemotherapy. Adjuvant chemotherapy with 5-FU with platinum and other agents is used especially for squamous cell cancer. However, it remains controversial whether this adds to survival time.

Side effects depend on the specific drug and the dose but include nausea, vomiting, poor appetite, hair loss, skin rash and itching, mouth and lip sores, diarrhea, and fatigue. These go away gradually during recovery between treatments or when it is over. Today there are many drugs to counteract nausea and some of the other side effects.

Radiation

In radiotherapy, high-energy rays kill cancer cells in the treated area only. The radiation may be from a machine outside the body (external radiation) or from radioactive materials placed in or near the tumor (internal radiation). A stent (plastic tube) may be inserted into the esophagus to keep it open during radiation therapy. This therapy may be used alone or combined with chemotherapy as primary treatment instead of surgery, especially if the size or location of the tumor (in the upper third of the esophagus) would make an operation difficult. It also may be combined with chemotherapy to shrink the tumor before surgery. Even if the tumor cannot be removed by surgery or destroyed entirely by radiation, this therapy often can help relieve pain and make swallowing easier.

Side effects depend mainly on the dose but may include a dry, sore mouth and throat; difficulty swallowing; swelling of the mouth and gums; dental cavities; fatigue; skin changes at the site of treatment; and loss of appetite.

Laser Therapy

Laser therapy is used to destroy cancerous tissue and relieve a blockage in the esophagus when the cancer cannot be removed by surgery. Relieving the blockage can help to reduce symptoms, especially problems swallowing. Short-term pain in the treatment area can be controlled with medication.

Photodynamic Therapy (PDT)   This is a type of laser therapy directed by endoscopy that uses drugs that are absorbed by the cancer cells. When exposed to a special light, the drugs become active and destroy the cancer cells. The doctor may use PDT to relieve symptoms of esophageal cancer, such as difficulty swallowing. PDT makes the skin and eyes highly sensitive to light for six weeks or longer after treatment. Other temporary effects may include coughing, trouble swallowing, abdominal pain, and painful breathing or shortness of breath.

Other Treatments

Some other treatments are used as palliative therapy for patients with inoperable cancer. These include endoscopic dilation and placing an expandable metal stent with endoscope. Palliative treatment with Photofrin is used when a tumor totally obstructs the esophagus. This is a photosensitizing method with endoscopic photodynamic therapy. There is some tumor response in a third of the patients according to clinical studies, and it may be better than thermal laser ablation.

Clinical Trials

Be sure to ask your doctor about clinical trials, and check the Web site of the National Institutes of Health and such cancer hospitals as Memorial Sloan Kettering in New York, M. D. Anderson in Houston, and Dana Farber in Boston.

Eating Well after Treatment

You may not feel like eating and also may have difficulty swallowing after esophageal cancer treatment. What's more, the nausea or dry mouth resulting from treatment makes it even more difficult. Foods may not taste the same as you remember, either, but you need to get sufficient calories and protein to maintain energy and strength.

After surgery you may receive nutrients intravenously or through a feeding tube until you are able to eat on your own. Once you are able to eat, several small meals and snacks throughout the day are more comfortable than eating three regular meals. If swallowing is difficult, you may be able to manage soft foods, or bland foods moistened with sauces or gravies. Puddings, yogurt, apple sauce, soups—even baby food—can be nourishing and easy to swallow. Your doctor will advise you to consult with a nutritionist following treatment.

Follow-up Care

Once you've been treated for cancer, you need periodic checkups for the rest of your life. This monitoring is necessary to find any recurring cancer early enough to treat it. If the cancer progresses or returns or if a new cancer develops, it can be treated as soon as possible. Checkups may include physical exams, X-rays, or lab tests. Between these follow-up appointments, be sure to report any changes to your doctor.

Other Disorders of the Esophagus

While you eat and your food is transported to your stomach, you are hardly aware of your esophagus if it is functioning normally. It operates on autopilot. Peristalsis and the lower esophageal sphincter (LES) keep everything moving smoothly. However, any impairment to the contractile force of your esophagus can create problems. A tumor or strictures could narrow the lumen—the hollow space. When the space is too narrow, contractile force is reduced. These are known as motility (motion) problems.

Other possible problems involve impacted food or a perforation.

Achalasia

Achalasia is a rare but classical esophageal motility disorder. The lower esophageal sphincter (LES) fails to relax during swallowing so there is no peristalsis in at least two thirds of the esophagus. This means that food is dropping down a chute, only to pile up at the end. Achalasia is caused by a motor neuron defect usually from some damage to the myenteric plexus, a network of nerve fibers and neuron cells in the digestive tract that coordinate the muscle contractions. In most cases of achalasia the nerve cells in the lower two-thirds of the esophagus and LES are abnormal. As a result, peristalsis is uncoordinated or weak and the LES fails to open.

The cause of achalasia is unknown, but it may be a degenerative disease of the nerves that supply the esophagus. Another theory is that it is caused by a virus, possibly herpes zoster, the same virus that causes shingles. Approximately 65 percent of people with this condition have autoantibodies against DARPP-32, a dopamine-carrying protein on the surface of myenteric plexus cells. It is associated with other diseases such as Parkinson's and Chagas's as well as familial syndromes such as All-grove's, familial achalasia, and hereditary ataxia. Achalasia can occur at any age, but it most often begins when people are in their thirties or forties. There is no gender or ethnic predilection, and it does not run in families. About two thousand new cases are diagnosed in the United States each year.

Jerome was only thirty, but he had a ten-year history of slowly progressive reflux symptoms when he noticed regurgitated food on his pillow at night. He also had severe halitosis, tightening chest pain, and he had lost fifteen pounds in the past year. A chest X-ray revealed a widening of the mediastinum, the center of his chest cavity, which allowed an "air-fluid" level behind his heart. An esophagram confirmed a lack of muscular tone in the esophagus, ending in a "bird beak" appearance on the X-ray. Endoscopy confirmed that his esophagus was dilated and filled with food. His hypertensive LES failed to relax, and there were changes throughout the wall of the esophagus. Manometry tests confirmed a lack of peristalsis. He was offered treatment by pneumatic dilatation or surgical myotomy. Because Jerome was only thirty and otherwise healthy, he was a good candidate for successful surgery for his achalasia. Jerome asked his doctor about the use of endoscopic botox injections to the LES. The botox therapy, however, would have been more appropriate in elderly patients who were not strong enough for surgery.

Symptoms

Symptoms of achalasia usually develop for most people between ages twenty-five and sixty, but it can occur even in children. The onset of symptoms—some similar to those of reflux disease—is gradual, and it may take years to progress. These include:

- difficulty swallowing solid food
- vomiting of undigested food
- chest pain, especially after meals
- coughing, especially at night when lying down
- difficulty swallowing liquids (later in the illness)
- weight loss (late)

Diagnosis of Achalasia

To confirm a diagnosis of achalasia, several tests can be done. We also need to rule out motion disorders of the esophagus such as spasm, scleroderma, stricture, or Schatzki's ring (see page 73).

Esophageal manometry   A thin tube is passed through your nose into your stomach. Pressure measurements are recorded while you drink sips of water as the tube is slowly withdrawn. People with achalasia have characteristic decreases in the force of peristaltic contractions, with elevated pressure readings at the LES. The LES also fails to relax.

Barium swallow (esophagraphy)   After swallowing barium, the lower esophagus, once dilated, fills with a "bird beak" appearance that can be seen on X-ray.

Chest X-ray   This is to check for a widened mediastinum, the space taken up by the dilated esophagus.

Endoscopy   Even if the results of manometry or esophagography suggest achalasia, endoscopy usually is done to rule out other diseases, such as infections or inflammatory conditions, cancer, and other disorders associated with achalasia.

See chapter 3 for more information about the tests.

Treating Achalasia

Medication is not very effective in treating achalasia, so therapy focuses on procedures that expand the esophageal lumen, mechanically or surgically.

Balloon (Pneumatic) Dilation

In this procedure a balloon is inserted and expanded inside the esophagus to make it wider. It can be tried again if it doesn't work the first time. The remission rate over a year with this procedure is 70 percent, and is widely thought to be the best initial treatment. The muscle fibers will be stretched, thus relieving the pressure that blocks easy passage of food into the stomach. Between 51 and 93 percent of people have relief of their symptoms for several years after this procedure. Repeat dilation may be needed for ongoing benefit. The chief risk of this procedure is rupture of the esophagus, which occurs in about 2 to 3 percent of patients and requires emergency surgery.

Myotomy

Known as the Heller method, this surgical technique is used to widen the LES opening and is 90 percent effective. Laparoscopic myotomy is performed with telescopic equipment through small incisions in the abdomen. Most people have good to excellent results. Even with older forms of myotomy, benefits have been observed for five years following surgery. In the past, surgery was reserved for those in whom balloon dilation was not successful. However, newer surgical techniques have led to improved outcomes with shorter hospital stays and lower risks.

Botulinum Toxin (Botox) Injection

This is an intramuscular injection into the LES. Tiny amounts of botox injected directly into the LES under endoscopic guidance paralyze and then relax the sphincter, allowing food to pass readily into the stomach. Botox is expensive, however, and its effects are relatively short-lived. It is effective in decreasing symptoms about a week after the injection and lasts about six months. Ninety percent of people will respond right away with only 65 percent still noticing swallowing difficulty at three months. However, after two years, nearly everybody relapses. Only 32 percent of people receiving this treatment were doing well after a year, compared to 70 percent of those receiving pneumatic dilation. Some will respond to another injection. It appears to be safe, but long-term effects have not been studied.

Medications

When these are called for, smooth-muscle dilators such as nitroglycerin or calcium channel blockers are used. Drugs that reduce LES pressure such as nifedipine (Adalat, Procardia) and nitroglycerin may be useful as adjuncts.

Carbonated Beverages

These often help loosen LES and may improve symptoms. The expanding carbon dioxide gas at body temperature may help push food through the LES.

Esophageal Spasm

Peristalsis is an unconscious, coordinated series of muscle contractions in the esophagus that moves food from your mouth to your stomach. If these contractions are no longer coordinated, or if they are too fast, or if all the muscles are moving at once, it not only hurts, it also does nothing to move food along. As a result, you can't swallow well, and food gets stuck. If it happens from eating hot or cold food, you may have a hypersensitive esophagus. While the condition does not lead to any long-term damage, the pain can be so disabling that it makes people afraid to eat and leads to loss of weight and being malnourished. Women are more likely than men to have esophageal spasms, but the cause is unknown.

Louise is twenty-nine and has been to a hospital emergency room many times during the past six months for episodes of chest pain. Typically, without warning, she experiences tightening chest pain that is unrelated to exercise but sometimes is related to drinking cold beverages. In the past, Louise has been under a psychiatrist's care for anxiety. A cardiac evaluation showed no problem, her blood tests and X-ray were normal, and an upper endoscopy was normal. However, esophageal manometry revealed that as much as 80 percent of her swallows are nonperistaltic—or simultaneous and often of high amplitude.

Treating Esophageal Spasm

No treatment for esophageal spasm works for everyone. A doctor may try several approaches before finding one that works. Sometimes the symptoms improve but never go away entirely. Dilatation (see page 38) can expand the esophagus. Nitrate medications such as nitroglycerin (the same as used to treat heart pain) and calcium channel blockers also are used but can cause nausea, constipation, and other side effects. Low doses of medications normally used for depression and antianxiety drugs also may help a hypersensitive esophagus but not without side effects. Nitrates can cause headaches and low blood pressure.

Hypocontracting Esophagus

Just as spasms and hypercontractions can cause problems and pain, a hypocontracting esophagus is working in slow motion. Usually this is diagnosed as a nonspecific esophageal motility disorder (NEMD). With manometry we can identify low-amplitude contractions or failed peristalsis in which the wave of contractions does not traverse the entire length of the esophagus. Sometimes this condition is associated with reflux esophagitis. Heartburn and acid regurgitation are more common than difficulty swallowing. H-2 agonists and proton pump inhibitors are used to treat it.

Esophageal Varices

Esophageal varices are dilated veins in the lower esophagus that usually are associated with advanced liver disease. They can cause bleeding and are potentially life-threatening. In the United States and other Western countries the primary cause is cirrhosis of the liver from alcohol abuse or hepatitis B (see page 159 for more on this).

Esophageal Diverticula

Any tubular organ can develop diverticula—sacs or pouches that protrude outward from the tube. These are more common in the colon (see page 220) but also can occur in the esophagus. Most esophageal diverticula occur in people in their seventies and eighties. While rare, esophageal diverticula usually are caused by a motility disorder in the esophagus such as spasm or achalasia.

The most common symptom is difficulty swallowing solids and even liquids. Food and secretions collect in these pouches and cause regurgitation of undigested food. (Some people find regurgitated food on their pillow when they wake up in the morning.) They can cause halitosis and coughing, too. When these sacs are in the upper esophagus and get very large, a mass in the neck sometimes can be seen.

Esophageal diverticula usually can be detected with a barium swallow and other tests. There is no treatment for esophageal diverticula, except to treat the underlying disorder.

Systemic Sclerosis (Scleroderma/CREST)

We don't know yet what causes scleroderma, but the course and severity of the disease vary widely. Excess collagen deposits in the skin and other organs produce external or internal symptoms—or both. You can see the results of this condition in pigment changes or ulcers on the skin. However, inside the body, changes may include fibrosis and degeneration of the heart, lungs, kidneys and gastrointestinal tract. The disease usually affects people thirty to fifty years old. Women are affected more often than men. Risk factors include occupational exposure to silica dust and polyvinyl chloride.

The CREST syndrome gets its name from the characterizations of scleroderma symptoms. The C is for calcinosis (calcium deposits); the R is for Raynaud's; the E is for the loss of muscle control of the esophagus;

the S is for sclerodactyly, a deformity of the skin of the fingers; and the T is for telangiectasia, small red spots on the skin of the fingers or face.

Because symptoms of CREST are just like those of any number of gastrointestinal conditions, your doctor will first have to rule out all the others to diagnose it. Symptoms include difficulty swallowing, heartburn or reflux disease, bloating after meals, shortness of breath, and weight loss, all indications of a host of other gastrointestinal conditions. Your doctor would have to look for other symptoms, such as tightness or thickening of your skin.

In most people, this disease is progressive. If the progression is slow, sometimes a remission occurs. If the disease affects only the skin, the probable outcome is better. When it affects internal organs, such as the gastrointestinal system, it leads to malabsorption of nutrients from the intestinal tract.

There is no treatment for this disease.

Perforated Esophagus

A perforated esophagus is a surgical emergency because a virulent internal infection can occur. Unless the perforation is high in the esophagus—in the neck area—it can kill you within twenty-four to forty-eight hours. Bacteria from the mouth and esophagus will spill inside the body and contaminate it. Secondary infection occurs rapidly from bacteria, gastric acid, and digestive enzymes and causes severe pain and erythema (reddened skin from irritated and congested small blood vessels). Pulmonary complications also may develop.

Chicken bones are the most common cause of perforated esophagus in adults. Holes in the esophagus also can result from an accidental injury such as when a doctor uses an endoscope to look in the esophagus or inserts a stomach tube through the nose to feed a person or to remove the contents of his or her stomach. Perforation can be caused by cancer, trauma, or corrosive esophagitis from acid or alkali ingestion. When reflux disease is not treated, it can create ulcers that eat through the wall of the esophagus, leaving a hole. Perforation can even happen spontaneously from severe vomiting known as Mallory-Weiss syndrome, which tears the lower esophagus.

Antibiotics and surgery are needed right away—it's a surgical emergency. An expanding esophageal mesh stent may be placed to bridge the tear, and the esophagus may heal itself. To locate the tear, doctors will do a CT scan or radiograph. A gastrograffin swallow is okay for the first study, but it misses 20 percent of perforations. It is critical to avoid aspiration of the gastrograffin, which would cause pulmonary edema, pneumonitis, and lead to death. A barium swallow is safe, but it is not effective with large tears.

Esophageal Infections

The esophagus can become infected from a variety of conditions. For example, the candida fungus, which causes oral thrush, a white coating, also can spread into the esophagus. Treatment is aimed at the underlying cause. Esophagitis with or without ulcers can develop inside the esophagus from candida, herpes simplex virus, cytomegalovirus, and, rarely, bacterial infections.

Candida esophagitis can be caused by antibiotics, treatment with radiation or chemotherapy, or AIDS. Malnutrition and alcoholism also can be contributing factors, as can advanced age. When the infection is not treated, white plaques lining the esophagus can become dense and thick and may ulcerate or hemorrhage and can cause mobility problems.

After candida, herpes simplex virus is the most common cause of infectious esophagitis. This condition occurs most commonly in AIDS patients but it also can be caused by medications or cancer treatment.

Depending upon the cause, esophageal infections are treated with medications such as antifungal agents or antiviral and other agents.

A Foreign Body in the Esophagus: The Steakhouse Syndrome and Schatzki's Ring

Children swallow parts of toys, and very commonly, coins. Usually these objects are removed if they are in the upper two-thirds of the esophagus. If they can't be removed without risk of tearing the esophagus, the child has to be watched for twelve hours. Most small foreign bodies pass spontaneously.

Adults, of course, don't put nonedible things in their mouth, but sometimes they accidentally swallow dentures or parts of eating utensils. The most common "foreign body" is probably food impaction, known as a food bolus (esophageal food bolus obstruction) and commonly called the steakhouse syndrome.

After swallowing a large mouthful, usually of inadequately chewed meat, chest pain that feels like a heart attack develops. This discomfort increases with swallowing, and is followed by retained salivary secretions, which, unlike a heart attack, lead to drooling. Most people arrive at the hospital with a receptacle under the mouth into which they are repeatedly spitting. At times these secretions will cause paroxysms of coughing, gagging, or choking.

If the stuck object is hard or sharp, such as a chicken bone, it also may cause a tear. As mentioned, chicken bones are the most common cause of esophageal perforation in adults. This is why Paul's coworkers rushed him to the hospital after he got severe chest pain after eating some Buffalo wings at a local restaurant. After several rounds of drinks, the chicken wings were passed around the table. In seconds, Paul, forty-eight, had pain beneath his breastbone. Although anxious, he was able to breathe and drink some water. Coughing, he went to the men's room to see if he could force himself to throw up and get rid of the stuck meat. That failed, so he was taken to the hospital emergency room, where a barium X-ray revealed the impacted food in the esophagus. A gastroenterologist performed an emergency upper endoscopy and extracted the impacted food. Further investigation, however, found that Paul had a Schatzki's mucosal ring just above a small hiatal hernia, and as a result, the lower part of his esophagus had narrowed. He later had a balloon dilation treatment to expand the space. However, part of Paul's problem was drinking enough to anesthetize his throat and upper esophagus, so he wasn't aware of not chewing his food properly.

While getting food stuck this way sometimes can result from intoxication, wearing dentures, or being too embarrassed to spit out a large piece of gristle, it is most often caused by some underlying esophageal problem.

People who experience these problems usually are over sixty and may have a benign stricture resulting from reflux esophagitis. Another abnormality is the Schatzki's ring, a mild narrowing of the lower esophagus caused by fibrous scar tissue. (A more severe scar tissue would be a stricture.) Some doctors believe that this tissue is present at birth and only causes problems as people age. However, most doctors believe it results from chronic reflux disease. Although the acid reflux may not be severe enough to cause heartburn, it may cause inflammation in the lower esophagus that eventually forms scar tissue. A Schatzki's ring is often detected during endoscopic tests for unrelated digestive complaints. However, most of the rings never cause problems and don't need therapy.

Most food particles and all liquids easily pass the ring, but larger pieces of solid food, such as steak or other meat, can get stuck at the ring. If you cannot get it unstuck by drinking water or vomiting, emergency treatment is called for.

Treating Esophageal Impaction

Meat impacted in the upper two-thirds of the esophagus is unlikely to pass and should be removed as soon as possible. Meat impacted in the lower third frequently does pass spontaneously, so it is safe to wait under medical observation up to twelve hours before extraction. Even if a meat bolus does not pass spontaneously, endoscopy still must be done later to assess the almost certain—80 to 90 percent—underlying pathology.

Your doctor will want a complete history and physical examination. If esophageal perforation is suspected, X-rays of your neck and chest will be taken to look for underlying respiratory conditions such as emphysema or pneumonia. If the food does not pass and you do not have access to a gastroenterologist with an endoscope, your doctor can do a manual extraction. Intravenous drugs will relax you and your pharynx. The doctor will push a tube through your mouth and esophagus until the obstruction is reached. Then, using a large aspiration syringe, he or she can apply suction and slowly withdraw it. If suction is maintained, the bolus will come up with the tubing. If that doesn't work, an endoscopist can use a flexible fiberoptic esophagoscope. Additional modes of therapy include use of drugs to relax the lower esophageal sphincter, but they are not as effective as intravenous glucagon.

When removal of the bolus is successful, medical follow-up should include a comprehensive evaluation of the esophagus. Therapy for Schatzki's ring is dilation, or stretching, of the ring to break it and prevent further episodes.

Treating the Underlying Rings or Webs

Rings and webs are the most common structural abnormalities in the esophagus. The terms often are used interchangeably. They don't cause many symptoms, but there is difficulty swallowing. Most are never noticed except during endoscopic examination.

A ring is a built-up layer of the esophageal lining. There are three types, but the most common is Schatzki's ring, usually located near the end of the esophagus and a hiatal hernia. Some scientists believe that this ring is a protective barrier against reflux disease. However, a common complication of this ring involves meat boluses.

If these rings do cause difficulty swallowing, you can modify your diet by eating soft food, cutting solid food into smaller pieces, and eating slowly and chewing thoroughly. Food impaction, particularly of meat products, is common with lower esophageal rings. Soft foods such as pasta and vegetables are less likely than meat to become lodged in the esophagus.

Even medications should be cut up. If a large pill would lodge in your esophagus, cut it into smaller pieces. Also drink at least eight ounces of liquid with the pills, and don't lie down for half an hour. Rings are generally treated by dilation (see page 38).

Chapter 5

The Stomach

THE STOMACH is a hollow, elastic sac shaped a bit like the letter J or a large kidney bean that fills and empties, digests and secretes. It sits in the upper abdomen just under the ribs and forms the widest part of the digestive tube. The upper part of the stomach—the fundus—connects to the esophagus (gastroesophageal junction) at a point known as the cardia. The lower part—the antrum—leads to the pyloric sphincter and the duodenum at the beginning of the small intestine.

Swallowed food collects in the fundus and moves to the antrum, which acts like a grinder, churning food back and forth until it is broken into smaller particles and sent into the duodenum. The stomach, like the heart, also has a pacemaker. This is like an electrical outlet that sets off the motion of the stomach muscles, causing them to contract. The pacemaker is in the upper part of the stomach but sets off the waves that go into the antrum and make it work. About three contractions occur every minute. This is much slower than the heart rate, but it does the job.

While the muscles in the wall of the stomach create a rippling motion that mixes and mashes the food, the juices made by peptic glands in the lining of the stomach help digest the food. Within three hours the food becomes liquid (called chyme) and moves into the small intestine where digestion continues. The pyloric sphincter opens to allow small quantities of food at a time to pass into the duodenum.

The stomach wall has four main layers. The serosa is the outer layer; the mucosa, the inner lining. Between these are two more layers: the muscularis and the submucosa. The surface of the mucosa is heavily folded and covered with numerous gastric pits that contain glands. Three to seven gastric glands open into the bottom of each of these small pits or indentations. These glands produce about six pints of gastric juice a day.

Deep in the glands are specialized cells that secrete acid and enzymes, all of which play an essential part in the digestive process. Pepsin is an enzyme that breaks down proteins into smaller units called polypeptides and peptides. Lipase breaks down a small proportion of fats into glycerol and fatty acids. Mucous-secreting cells protect the inner layer of the stomach. Hydrochloric acid is produced to assist the action of pepsin and also to kill certain bacteria. Stomach acid is more potent than battery acid.

Stomach conditions discussed in this chapter include:

- dyspepsia
- gastritis
- duodenal and gastric ulcers
- benign gastric tumors
- stomach cancer
- gastroparesis
- foreign bodies in the stomach

Dyspepsia, Gastritis, and Ulcers

Indigestion, gastritis, and ulcers are the most common afflictions of the stomach, a large, hollow organ that is also a very complex system of muscles, nerves, and chemicals.

Dyspepsia

As many as 40 percent of the people in the United States have dyspepsia, another word for indigestion, but only about 5 percent go to a doctor to treat it. Dyspepsia is a symptom of a disease such as gastric or duodenal ulcer or it can be a functional disorder rather than an organic disease. This means there is nothing physically wrong with the digestive organs, but they are not functioning properly. For example, the stomach muscles, or the system of nerves that serve the entire length of the gastrointestinal tract, may not be in synch. Both sensory and motor nerves are involved, so if the small intestine is stretched to accommodate the passage of food, it may give rise to sensory signals that are sent to the spinal cord and brain, where they are perceived as painful. Estrogen also may have some role, because some women say dyspepsia is worse during their menstrual cycle. Other gastrointestinal conditions, as well as diabetes, thyroid disease, and kidney disease also have been associated with dyspepsia. Medications such as NSAIDs and antibiotics cause it in some patients.

Functional dyspepsia is a chronic condition that lasts for years, although it may come and go or be more frequent or severe for weeks, months, or days. We don't know why it fluctuates, but it causes pain, discomfort, and other symptoms in the upper abdomen. Some sufferers may have *H. pylori*, but even if the bacteria are wiped out with antibiotics, the symptoms often remain.

People with functional dyspepsia usually have a relapsing condition. In an early fifteen-year study in a rural community, 65 percent of those with dyspepsia at the beginning of the study had the same symptoms three years later. A more recent study in the United States in 1998 found that 86 percent of those studied had it after twelve to twenty months. A British study the same year found that 75 percent of people had it after two years.

Symptoms and Diagnosis of Dyspepsia

Symptoms of dyspepsia include pain above the navel; belching; nausea (and perhaps vomiting); feeling full after a small amount of food; and sometimes abdominal swelling, known in medical terms as "meteorism." Symptoms most often occur after eating. Even though we talk about dyspepsia as a condition, it is really a symptom in itself.

Diagnosis of dyspepsia is based on symptoms and by ruling out other medical or psychiatric causes. The differential diagnosis of dyspepsia falls into four major categories: chronic peptic ulcer disease, reflux disease, a malignancy, or functional dyspepsia. To rule out all else, tests may include an upper GI endoscopy, upper GI series, small-bowel series, and barium enema X-ray of the colon (see chapters 2 and 3). A breath test can rule out the presence of bacterial overgrowth of the small intestine, which also can cause dyspepsia.

Treating Functional Dyspepsia

Because it is a functional disorder rather than an organic disease, functional dyspepsia can be difficult to treat. No mechanical problems can be targeted, so we can only treat the symptoms. For example, nausea can be suppressed with medications, but that won't get at the cause of the condition. Treatment approach depends on the person's age and symptoms, as well as on how long he or she has had those symptoms.

A multifaceted treatment, similar to the type used for irritable bowel disease, another functional disease, is the most successful. This includes diet and lifestyle changes as well as medications.

In recent years there has been more research focusing on visceral (hyper) sensitivity and visceral reflexes, because it is thought that some people have altered visceral perception, or internal cognition. There is no optimal treatment, however.

Education

By keeping a record of symptoms, you can begin to see patterns or learn just when the symptoms are caused by certain foods or situations. Learning how and when dyspepsia occurs helps you learn how to stay comfortable and avoid symptoms.

Diet and Lifestyle

Although certain foods may aggravate symptoms of functional dyspepsia, food is not the cause. Nevertheless, some people feel better if they eliminate foods that seem to bring on symptoms, such as:

- fatty foods such as French fries and fried chicken
- sausages, cold cuts, and meat that is highly marbled with fat, as found in many cuts of beef and pork
- raw foods with strong flavors, such as radishes
- citrus fruits such as orange, lime, lemon, and grapefruit
- acidic foods such as tomatoes, pickles, and vinegar dressings
- foods that are highly spiced with chili pepper and other seasonings common to Mexican and Asian cuisines
- coffee, tea, and caffeinated sodas
- alcohol

Lactose intolerance is often blamed for functional dyspepsia but may not be the cause. Eating more small meals rather than a few large ones prevents the stomach from extending. If you smoke, try to quit. Cigarette smoking is a known irritant of the stomach.

Medication

Prokinetic and antispasmodic medications are successful in some cases. Smooth-muscle relaxants and promotility drugs are most often used to control symptoms of dyspepsia. Sometimes taking antacids such as Mylanta or Maalox an hour before eating and at bedtime helps.

Drugs that are used for irritable bowel syndrome also are successful in treating dyspepsia. These include amitriptyline, clonidine, sumatriptan, octreotide, and fedotozine. Drugs such as atropine or hyoscine are nonspecific smooth-muscle relaxants. They reduce severe episodes of pain arising from gut spasm, but they have adverse effects on the bladder, eyes, and salivary glands. Tricyclic antidepressants also seem to relieve symptoms, whether or not the patient is depressed. A blocking agent called metoclopramide increases the movements or contractions of the stomach.

Always avoid aspirin and NSAIDs in treating dyspepsia.

Gastritis

Gastritis is an inflammation of the stomach lining. It is not a single disease, but a condition that can be caused by long-term use of aspirin and other nonsteroidal anti-inflammatory drugs (NSAIDs), alcohol abuse, or bacterial infection such as the common *Helicobacter pylori (H. pylori)*. Severe infections or burns from the ingestion of a corrosive substance also can damage the stomach lining. Less common causes are some autoimmune disorders such as pernicious anemia, or chronic reflux of bile and pancreatic fluids from the duodenum. Gastritis can be caused by anything that might cause the stomach to produce excessive acid or weaken the mucous membrane stomach lining, especially medications or poor blood supply to the mucosa. In some people extreme physical stress or the development of liver failure can cause gastritis. When the inflammation is in the stomach we call it gastritis, and duodenitis when it's in the duodenum. Gastritis is not generally a serious condition, but sometimes it can cause significant bleeding. If it continues long enough it can ulcerate the stomach lining. Gastritis can come on suddenly or may be chronic and develop gradually over time.

Barbara, fifty-five, complained of a burning sensation after she ate. She had been using nonsteroidal anti-inflammatory drugs for arthritis pain and also antacids to relieve the burning pain. The burning got worse and she noticed some darkening of her bowel movements (a sign of gastrointestinal bleeding) as well as abdominal tenderness on the left side. Endoscopic examination and biopsy revealed a classic case of gastritis. Under the microscope (or biopsy) pathologists describe four major forms of gastritis:

- superficial gastritis, the initial sign of the condition
- gastritis associated with *H. pylori* infection
- acute gastritis, the most serious, usually found in seriously ill patients or those using NSAIDs; erosions are caused by medication effect or stress to the stomach lining

• Atrophic gastritis, from the wearing away of the stomach lining; this may predispose to gastric cancer

Symptoms and Diagnosis of Gastritis

Abdominal pain and upset are the most common symptoms of gastritis; others include bloating or a feeling of fullness, nausea and vomiting, belching, or a burning pain in the upper abdomen. Signs of blood in the stool, or vomiting blood, may indicate bleeding in the stomach that needs immediate medical attention.

Gastritis is diagnosed with upper gastrointestinal endoscopy (see chapter 3). Using the lighted tube with a camera on the end, the doctor can see if the stomach lining is inflamed. A tissue sample can be removed for biopsy to confirm if *H. pylori* is present or to rule out other possible causes. Blood tests can reveal whether loss of blood has caused anemia. A stool test also checks for signs of bleeding and may be used to detect the shedding of the *H. pylori* from the stomach lining. This is done with a frozen stool specimen.

Treating Gastritis

Gastritis should be treated if there are symptoms. If *H. pylori* is present, treatment must include an antibiotic regimen. (There's more about the *H. pylori* later in this chapter.) Because stomach acid irritates the inflammation, medications can reduce stomach acid, relieve symptoms, and promote healing. Abstaining from alcohol and certain spicy or acidic foods also can relieve the problem.

Ulcers

Peptic ulcers develop in the stomach and duodenum. The condition of having gastric or duodenal ulcers is called peptic ulcer disease (PUD), for the digestive enzyme pepsin. An ulcer is a break or chronic sore in the lining of the stomach or duodenum. It can form in any area exposed to gastric acid and pepsin. Modern drugs heal virtually all benign peptic ulcers, but they can come back if *H. pylori* is present and not eliminated. (On occasion, gastric ulcers can be malignant.) *H. pylori* infection and use of NSAIDs are the primary causes of ulcers, which are one of the most common conditions of the gastrointestinal tract. About 10 percent of Americans have ulcers. However, ulcers are not always easy to diagnose because there may be no symptoms or only vague pain. Although men and women are equally vulnerable to gastritis, about twice as many men develop ulcers.

Ulcers occur only in the presence of stomach acid, but they are not caused just by excessive quantities of acid. People who produce low levels of acid sometimes get them, while others who produce large amounts of acid may be ulcer-free. Distortion of the balance between stomach acid secretion and protective mucus is the likely cause. When the mucous lining of the stomach is not adequate, even a small amount of acid can cause an ulcer. Normally, the stomach maintains a balance between protective factors such as blood flow, mucous and bicarbonate secretions, and harmful factors such as too much acid secretion or pepsin.

Drinking alcohol and smoking probably do not directly cause ulcers, but those habits can contribute to their formation.

Stomach Ulcers

About 70 percent of stomach ulcers are from *H. pylori* and the rest from the use of NSAIDs or aspirin for arthritis or musculoskeletel pain. Stomach ulcers usually cause pain in the upper middle of the abdomen (epigastrium) or just below the rib cage on the left side. Eating—especially certain foods—may aggravate stomach ulcers at first, but the burning sensation subsides as the food begins to buffer the stomach acid. Stomach ulcers occur more often in people over forty, usually because of the higher use of aspirin and NSAIDs to treat arthritis.

Duodenal Ulcers

These usually occur in people between twenty and forty, probably because younger people produce more acid. At least 90 percent are caused by *H. pylori*. Burning pain from these ulcers may be felt in the epigastrium or a little to the right. Eating often relieves pain. Duodenal ulcers are four times more common than gastric ulcers, with a lifetime prevalence of 10 percent for men and 5 percent for women, although the gender gap is closing.

There are 200,000 to 400,000 new cases of duodenal ulcers annually in the United States, compared to 87,500 new cases of gastric ulcers.

Ulcers Caused by *H. pylori*

H. pylori is the leading cause of PUD. These bacteria colonize in the deep layers of the mucosal lining of the stomach. While acid kills most bacteria, *H. pylori* can exist in an acid environment because it produces an enzyme called urease that synthesizes ammonia. Ammonia neutralizes the acid and allows *H. pylori* to thrive.

Once established, *H. pylori* will set up shop in your stomach for life. It lives in the mucous layer, producing chemicals and proteins that damage the lining. Most infected people develop gastritis but otherwise manage to live in harmony with the bug. Only a minority get ulcers or cancer, but it's not clear why some do and some don't. There may be other risk factors, such as genetic predisposition or a particularly virulent strain of the bug.

Cigarette smoking also is believed to play a role in *H. pylori* infection because of its negative effect on the mucosal lining of the stomach. People who smoke tend to have frequent or recurrent ulcers that are more resistant to treatment.

It is estimated that 60 percent of Americans over sixty have *H. pylori* lurking in their stomach lining. More than 80 percent of adult Japanese, Latin Americans, Asians, and Africans are infected with *H. pylori*.

We don't know exactly how one gets infected, but it probably happens from contact with an infected person's vomit, or by sharing foods or utensils. Spread among family members is not uncommon. If you have the *H. pylori* infection, then your family, especially your spouse and young children, are likely to get it. Once infected, there's a 15 percent chance of developing an ulcer. This infection puts you at higher risk for stomach cancers. The World Health Organization declared *H. pylori* a Class 1 carcinogen. In childhood, infection is transmitted by the fecal oral route, but after age five the risk is reduced because older children generally have better hygiene. In some parts of world *H. pylori* is in the water supply. The poor are at higher risk because of crowded living conditions and poor hygiene in childhood. Today the bacteria along with stomach cancer seem to be dying out in developed countries but increasing in underdeveloped countries.

There may be a genetic reason for vulnerability to this bacteria. A bacterial gene called cagA is associated with severe gastritis, gastric ulcer, and gastric cancer as well as lymphoma.

Ulcers Caused by NSAIDs

Many older people take aspirin to prevent a heart attack, or they take NSAIDs such as Motrin and Aleve for arthritis pain. These drugs erode the stomach lining and account for about 25 percent of gastric ulcers. The greatest risk of developing an ulcer occurs during the first three months of NSAID use. After that, the risk decreases but is still present. Ulcers induced by NSAIDs are usually silent, meaning they cause no symptoms until they begin to bleed.

Aspirin and NSAIDs block the production of the hormonelike substance prostaglandin by interfering with the enzyme cyclooxygenase or COX, which is needed to make prostaglandin. Prostaglandin stimulates mucus and bicarbonate production in the stomach. Mucus protects the stomach lining from acid and bicarbonate neutralizes stomach acid. COX inhibitors such as Celebrex and other new arthritis medications prevent this interference.

Complications of ulcers include perforation, obstruction, hemorrhage, and gastric cancer (if you have a gastric ulcer). The risk of cancer is about 2 percent in the first three years. A risk factor related to the *H. pylori* infection is atrophic gastritis, which increases the risk of cancer. *H. pylori* infection is also associated with gastric lymphoma (known as MALT lymphoma because it starts in the mucosa-associated lymphoid tissue). When ulcers are bleeding, hospitalization is often required.

Symptoms and Diagnosis of Ulcers

The primary symptom of an ulcer is a burning pain in the mid or upper left side of the abdomen that may radiate to the back. It usually occurs an hour or more after eating. Sometimes it is relieved by antacids or by vomiting. A sudden onset of symptoms could mean that an ulcer has perforated. Bleeding is more likely in older patients and may cause anemia and fatigue.

Breath tests and stool tests can identify the presence of *H. pylori*, but endoscopic testing still is needed to view the stomach lining. A complete blood count evaluates any blood loss, and a blood test determines the presence of *H. pylori* antibodies. Stool tests would also determine any hidden loss of blood and could detect the shedding of *H. pylori*. A chest X-ray may be helpful to see if there is free abdominal air that would be a sign of perforation. (The patient would be ill.) If the ulcer is not caused by *H. pylori* or NSAIDs, diagnostic testing must rule out all other possibilities, such as pancreatitis, inflammatory bowel disease, or gastric cancer. Ulcers usually are not malignant, however.

Treating Ulcers

The goal of ulcer treatment is to relieve the discomfort and heal the stomach lining. Medications always are used so that the ulcer doesn't get worse and perforate, bleed, or obstruct. There are four types of drugs used in ulcer treatment: antacids to neutralize stomach acid; sucralfate to protectively coat the ulcer; histamine blockers; and proton pump inhibitors (PPIs) to inhibit acid production. Most patients respond to PPIs faster than they do to antacids, which may be okay for mild cases.

For ulcers caused by NSAIDs, the preferred treatment is to stop use of those medications and treat the ulcers with H-2 blockers or PPIs. There are many new drugs for arthritis pain less likely to cause ulcers or gastritis. Ask your doctor which ones are best for you.

Treating H. pylori

For ulcers caused by *H. pylori*, treatment will take longer. Getting rid of *H. pylori* is a long, complicated process involving use of antibiotics, several treatment regimens, and follow-up treatment. Some *H. pylori* bugs have developed resistance to certain antibiotics. To complicate matters, treatment doesn't guarantee you won't get another ulcer, even though you are no longer infected.

Short-term, low-dose, triple-therapy regimens of PPIs and two antibiotics are the current gold standard therapy for cure of *H. pylori* infection. These consist of multiple drugs combined into one package. The American College of Gastroenterology, specialists in treating ulcers, no longer recommends two-drug regimens since they are not as effective as other treatment regimens. The four-drug regimens taken for two weeks are effective, too, but are complicated to take.

Problems with patient compliance and the development of antibiotic resistance are the two most important factors to consider when choosing a regimen.

Louis is a thirty-four-year-old accountant who has had stomach pain from recurrent duodenal ulcers since he was a teenager, although there is no history of ulcers in his family. Over the years he has tried to relieve his symptoms with antacids, and he had good results from treatment with H-2 receptor agonists. He has never had any bleeding or perforation. He used to be a heavy smoker but he quit a year ago. Nevertheless, Louis's recurrent symptoms are quite severe. A biopsy revealed Louis has a large ulcer and moderate chronic active gastritis, and *H. pylori* was present. Treatment of his condition included plans to use antibiotics to eradicate *H. pylori*.

Acid Suppression Therapy

Antacids such as Maalox or Mylanta may control ulcer pain when properly used, along with changes in diet and lifestyle, but H-2 blockers are much more effective.

H-2 blockers usually are the first medications used to treat ulcers. They are available without prescription and provide symptomatic relief. These medications block histamine, a natural chemical in your body that stimulates stomach acid secretion. They prevent the histamine from attaching to your stomach cells that make acid. Over-the-counter H-2 blockers include:

- Pepcid AC
- Tagamet HB
- Zantac 75
- Axid AR

Carafate sometimes is used for short-term management of ulcers caused by NSAIDs once the NSAIDs have been discontinued. Carafate exudes an adhesive substance that protects the stomach lining against peptic acids and bile salts.

Proton Pump Inhibitors

Proton pump inhibitors (PPIs) attack the problem another way. They block the production of stomach acid altogether by shutting down a system in the stomach known as the proton pump. These drugs are very safe and more effective than H-2 blockers. In combination with other drugs, they also are used to treat the *H. pylori* infection of recurring stomach ulcers. You need a doctor's prescription for these drugs, except for one type of Prilosec, which was approved for over-the-counter sale in 2003. PPIs include:

- Prilosec
- Prevacid
- AcipHex
- Protonix
- Nexium
- Rapinex

PPIs come in pill and powder form, and one type can be injected intra-venously in the hospital. Intravenous PPIs are designed for patients who cannot take oral therapy, such as those in intensive care hospital units. Most people take these drugs for a month or two, but some may need to take them longer. Long-term treatment is safe and effective when the patient is monitored by a physician.

Who should not take PPIs?   If you have liver or kidney problems, or are pregnant or breast-feeding, then your doctor may want to limit your use of PPIs. If you take other medications you also need to be careful of interactions with PPIs. Don't use any other drugs, including any herbal remedies you may use without prescription, before talking with your doctor. If you take medications for epilepsy and prevention of blood clots, the effect of these drugs may be increased when you also take a proton pump inhibitor. Antifungal drugs may not be absorbed as well if you are using PPIs. The breakdown of Valium (diazepam) may be blocked by some of the PPIs.

Side effects   PPIs generally don't cause problems, but there are some side effects, including diarrhea, constipation, gas, abdominal pain, nausea, and headaches. In rare cases, they may cause allergic reactions such as itching, dizziness, muscle pain, or blurred vision. In some people long-term use can lead to stomach infections because stomach acid helps kill microscopic bacteria in the stomach—and the PPI stops acid production. If you notice tarry stools or you vomit, call your doctor right away. These are signs of intestinal bleeding.

Follow-up care   If you must take PPIs for long periods, you may need to have a periodic blood test to monitor your serum gastrin level and vitamin B_{12} level. (See chapter 4 for more information on these drugs and on vitamin B_{12} deficiency.) You also may need an upper endoscopy every two to three years. Visit your doctor in two to six weeks to evaluate the effectiveness of the treatment.

Benign Gastric Tumors and Stomach Cancer

An assortment of growths can sprout from the layers of the stomach wall. And since the advent of endoscopic testing, more of these benign growths have been discovered, whether or not there are symptoms. Small tumors usually cause no symptoms, but larger ones can ulcerate and bleed, causing anemia. Large tumors also can obstruct the digestive process and cause nausea, vomiting, and a feeling of fullness. If these growths ulcerate, they cause pain similar to that of a peptic ulcer. Symptomic gastric polyps should be removed when they are detected.

Judy, sixty-two, had intermittent nausea and vomiting for four months. Upper gastrointestinal endoscopy revealed a pedunculated central gastric polyp, causing intermittent obstruction in the gastric outlet.

(Polyps are either pedunculated, sticking up like a pimple, or sessile, having a flattened ridge shape.) The polyp was removed with snare electrocautery. Biopsy showed that she did not have *H. pylori* or cancer but did have gastritis. After a twelve-week course of proton pump inhibitor (PPI) therapy, a follow-up endoscopy showed complete healing with no remnants of the polyp. For the past eight months Judy has been symptom-free.

Polyps

Hyperplastic polyps are the most common type found in the stomach and vary in location and size. Most are smaller than two centimeters, about the size of a pencil eraser. Even though they are benign, they may be accompanied by atrophic gastritis, which predisposes the stomach mucous lining to malignant transformation. People with Menetrier disease often have multiple hyperplastic polyps. This disease of the stomach is characterized by giant hypertrophy of the stomach lining and cystic changes. A giant hypertrophy is large coiled folds that resemble polyps in the inner wall of the stomach. Enlarged gastric folds and an overall increase in the mucosal thickness occur. Acid secretion is low. It is a rare disease associated with protein loss that occurs most often in people over fifty. A wide variety of symptoms occur, including weight loss, abdominal pain and nausea, diarrhea, and gastrointestinal bleeding. Symptoms often develop for decades before they are discovered.

Adenomatous polyps usually are solitary tubular lesions in the antrum (lower stomach). They do have cells that are associated with stomach cancer, and this association is greatest when the polyp is larger than two centimeters in diameter.

Inflammatory fibroid polyps tend to become large and cause obstruction, so they are usually removed.

In some people there is a genetic predisposition to get stomach polyps. Such polyposis syndromes include juvenile polyps, familial polyposis syndrome, and Peutz-Jeghers syndrome. Fundic gland polyps contain microcysts and are common in familial polyposis syndrome.

Cysts and Tumors

Leiomyas are benign and are the most common smooth-muscle tumor of the stomach. They can arise from any part of the muscle of the stomach, cause obstruction, ulcerate, and hemorrhage. Leiomyas are now classified as a type of gastrointestinal stomach tumor or GIST tumor (see page 99).

Cystic tumors are the most common benign stomach cysts. They develop when a mucous-secreting gland is blocked. The secretions are trapped inside so the cyst grows and eventually causes obstruction. They need to be removed.

Diagnosis of Polyps

Many tumors are found incidentally during endoscopic procedures for other reasons. A tumor, polyp, or cyst may grow to a large enough mass that it can be felt by a doctor during a physical examination. It also may be tender to the touch. Naturally, a correct diagnosis can be done only after other things are ruled out, such as gastric ulcers, cancer, or gastric varices (enlarged blood vessels).

Treating Polyps

Endoscopic ultrasound is an effective way to locate the growth. Because the layers of the stomach wall are deep, endoscopic biopsies can be misleading. Gastric polyps can be removed (snared) endoscopically and cauterized if they are small. Larger polyps need to be removed operatively, and resection of the stomach may be necessary for multiple polyps. Small tumors can be treated with wide local excision of the surrounding stomach wall.

Stomach Cancer

The number of stomach cancer deaths in the United States has dropped dramatically in the past sixty years. Nevertheless, it is still a serious disease that affects about twenty-four thousand people each year and is the seventh-leading cause of cancer death here. In the rest of the world, gastric cancer is the second most common cause of cancer-related death. Many Asian countries, including Korea, China, Taiwan, and Japan, have very high rates. Stomach cancer remains difficult to cure in Western countries because most patients don't get it diagnosed until it is advanced. In Japan, however, a rigorous system of screening detects the cancer in its early stages, when it can be cured.

Also called gastric cancer, it can develop in any part of the stomach and spread along the stomach wall into the esophagus or small intestine. The most likely places for it to spread outside the stomach are the liver, pancreas, and colon. However, lungs and lymph nodes above the collarbone also are targets, as are the ovaries in women. Doctors cannot explain why one person gets it and another does not but some people are more likely to develop this cancer. Its demographic incidence is as follows:

- It is found most often in people over fifty-five.
- Men get it twice as often as women.
- It is more common in black people than whites.
- It is more common in Japan, Korea, parts of Eastern Europe, and Latin America than it is in the United States.

Some studies suggest that *H. pylori*, which causes stomach inflammation and ulcers, may be a risk factor for stomach cancer. Chronic infection with *H. pylori* in some susceptible people causes a change in the lining of the stomach to resemble the small intestine (intestinal melaplasia). As with Barrett's esophagus (see page 60), this type of change increases the risk of cancer, although it is not as great as with Barrett's. If this change is discovered, ask your doctor about having periodic endoscopic screenings.

Research also shows that people who have had stomach surgery or have pernicious anemia or gastric atrophy are at increased risk. Gastric atrophy shrinks and weakens the stomach muscles. The peptic glands also may shrink, resulting in lack of digestive juices.

Certain dusts and fumes in the workplace have also been linked to stomach cancer, and many scientists believe that cigarette smoking increases the risk.

Diet is suspected of being a risk factor for stomach cancer. Smoked meats, pickled vegetables, and excessive dietary salt increase the risk of stomach cancer. Preservative-laden lunch meats and hot dogs, as well as charcoal-broiled foods, produce nitrosamines that may cause cancer. High rates of stomach cancer are found in regions where people eat many foods that are preserved by drying, smoking, salting, or pickling.

H. pylori is responsible for most cases involving the bottom half of the stomach (antrum). In the fundus and near the esophagus, it is not usually related. *H. pylori* also can cause other forms of stomach cancer, such as non-Hodgkins lymphoma of the stomach. Also, some people are genetically predisposed to this cancer.

When stomach cancer is detected early, it can be cured. Unfortunately, there is no universal screening for this cancer. Most people do not discover it until it is advanced and more difficult to treat. If you have many family members with this cancer, get tested for it periodically. It can run in families because of genetic susceptibility or the same early infection with *H. pylori*.

Robert's cancer was not discovered until he had a prominent swollen lymph node near his neck. At sixty-seven Robert was referred to a gastroenterologist because he complained of feeling too full to eat and he had lost weight and had chronic bad breath. Tests revealed he was anemic and was bleeding internally. An upper endoscopy revealed the stomach cancer, and surgery showed it had spread to his lymph nodes, including the one near his neck. After surgery, Robert began a course of chemotherapy that kept his cancer at bay for some time.

Symptoms of Stomach Cancer

It is hard to find stomach cancer in its early stage because there often are no symptoms. When the symptoms do occur, they can be vague, and people often ignore them. Symptoms usually arrive late because of the large capacity of the stomach. Anyone who feels full after eating a small amount should have an upper gastrointestinal endoscopy to rule out cancer. Some symptoms include:

- indigestion or a burning sensation like heartburn
- discomfort or pain in the abdomen
- nausea and vomiting
- diarrhea or constipation
- bloating of the stomach after meals
- loss of appetite
- weakness and fatigue
- vomiting blood or passing blood in the stool

These symptoms also are typical of any number of other gastrointestinal conditions, so they all need to be ruled out.

Diagnosis and Staging of Stomach Cancer

Early diagnosis can be achieved if early warning signals such as bleeding are caught. If you are over fifty, an annual fecal blood test can discover any internal bleeding. If a colonoscopy then proves negative, an upper endoscopic investigation should be done. Most of this bleeding will be caused by gastritis or an ulcer, but it also may be caused by cancer.

Once cancer is identified, it is staged by scanning the body with CT or ultrasound. This will guide treatment and determine if the cancer has spread, and if so,where. Staging cannot be complete until after surgery, when nearby lymph nodes and organs can be tested.

The 1997 American Joint Committee on Cancer issued a cancer staging manual that presents the TNM classification system for staging gastric cancer:

Primary Tumor

TX = primary tumor (T) cannot be assessed

TO = no evidence of primary tumor

Tis = carcinoma in situ

T1 = tumor invading the submucosa

T2 = tumor invading the stomach wall muscle

T3 = tumor has penetrated the wall without invading adjacent structures

T4 = tumor has invaded adjacent structures

There are additional staging labels for regional and distant metastases, as well as ways to chart the pattern of spread.

Treating Stomach Cancer

Stomach cancer treatment depends on the size and location of the tumor, the stage of the disease, and the patient's general health. Because treatment decisions are complex, it is a good idea to get a second opinion. In fact, medical insurance companies often require it.

Treatment may include surgery (gastrectomy), chemotherapy, and/or radiation therapy. There are new approaches to treatment, such as biological therapy. Clinical trials usually test various combination therapies. Ask your doctor if you are eligible for any of these clinical trials.

Surgery: Gastrectomy

Stomach surgery—gastrectomy—removes part or all of the stomach as well as a margin of disease-free tissue around the cancer area. Lymph nodes near the tumor are taken out to be tested for cancer cells to determine if the disease has spread. There is an extensive lymphatic network around the stomach and the cancer is aggressive, so most surgeons maintain a margin around the tumor of at least five centimeters to assure that they get it all. The extent of lymph node removal remains somewhat controversial. Many studies show that nodal involvement means a poor prognosis, so surgeons are more aggressive about taking out lymph nodes. The remaining part of the stomach is reconnected to the esophagus and the small intestine. If the entire stomach is removed, the esophagus is connected directly to the small intestine.

For a few days after a gastrectomy, activities are limited so patient can heal. Intravenous feeding is necessary until liquids and soft foods can be ingested. If the entire stomach has been removed, the body can no longer absorb vitamin B$_{12}$, so regular injections are needed to put that vital nutrient directly into the blood stream. Some foods always will be difficult to digest following a gastrectomy, and for some people the taste of food changes forever.

After a gastrectomy, bile in the small intestine may back up into the remaining part of the stomach or into the esophagus. This causes an upset stomach, but medications may prevent that.

The Dumping Syndrome   When food and liquid enter the small intestine too quickly, it can cause cramps, nausea, diarrhea, and dizziness shortly after eating. This is the dumping syndrome. It can be prevented by eating several small meals throughout the day; eating foods high in protein; and avoiding foods high in sugar, which make the symptoms worse. Drinking with meals is discouraged so that less fluid enters the small intestine. Medications can help prevent the dumping syndrome. Symptoms usually go away within a year, but for some they may be permanent.

Chemotherapy

Chemotherapy treatment after surgery has a better chance of increasing survival than does radiotherapy. Treatment with chemotherapy kills cancer cells throughout the body, but it also kills many good cells while doing its job. This is what causes so many side effects. Chemotherapy is often given before surgery to shrink the stomach tumor. It is used after surgery as adjuvant therapy to destroy any remaining cancer cells. Doctors also are testing anticancer drugs put directly into the abdomen (intraperitoneal chemotherapy). The most widely studied drug regimen is 5-fluorouracil (5-FU), doxorubicin, and mitomycin-C.

Most chemotherapy drugs are given by injection in the doctor's office or a hospital as an outpatient procedure. Some are taken orally. Chemotherapy drugs are often used in combination. Sometimes several drugs are tried before the most effective one is identified. Chemotherapy is usually given in cycles, with a treatment followed by a recovery period before the next treatment.

Always ask your doctor what drugs you are getting, what the goal is, what the side effects are, how long treatment will last, and how you will know if it is working. During cancer treatment, periodic CT scans are done to find out if the cancer is shrinking or growing.

Side effects of chemotherapy include loss of hair, increased vulnerability to infections, nausea and vomiting, bruising, loss of energy, and mouth sores. Medications combat some of these side effects, but every individual reacts differently to the chemotherapy as well as to the side effects of medications.

Radiation

Radiation (radiotherapy) is local therapy that affects only the cells within its range. It is used after surgery to destroy any remaining cells in the area. When it cannot be used as a cure, radiation is used as palliative therapy to relieve pain. This treatment is done in the hospital, usually for five days a week over a period of five to six weeks.

In some clinical trials, radiation is being used during surgery to see if intraoperative radiotherapy shows promise. This allows for a high dose to be given in a single fraction while in the operating room so that other nearby critical structures can be avoided.

Radiation of the abdomen may cause nausea, vomiting, and diarrhea. Some medications and diet changes can relieve these problems. The skin of the abdomen may become tender, dry and red, and perhaps itchy. Wear loose clothing that doesn't rub, and ask your doctor to recommend a lotion or cream to combat the dry skin. Radiation makes you tired, so although you may go to work and have a normal day, it's important to take naps and get plenty of rest.

Biological Therapy

Biological therapy (immunotherapy) helps the immune system attack and destroy the cancer cells. It also may help the body recover from some of the side effects of other treatments. This is being studied in clinical trials in combination with other treatments to try to prevent the recurrence of stomach cancer.

Another use of biological therapy is to help restore a patient's blood cell levels during chemotherapy. This is called colony-stimulating factors.

Side effects of biotherapy may include flulike symptoms, weakness, nausea, and vomiting. These can be severe and most patients are kept in the hospital for this type of therapy.

There are many clinical trials to find the best ways to treat stomach cancer. Talk with your doctor to find out if you are eligible for any of these trials. For information, contact the National Cancer Institute (see the appendix).

Other Gastric Malignancies

There are a few rare gastric cancers:

MALT Lymphoma (Non-Hodgkins Lymphoma)

MALT means mucosa-associated lymphoma tissue. Generally the digestive tract is not associated with lymphoid tissue, except for small collections of white blood cells, B-lymphocytes, that may accumulate in response to *H. pylori* infections or as the result of autoimmune conditions. When the growth of these lymphocytes continues through infection, a malignant cell may arise and replace the normal tissue. These lymphomas, growing from the mucosa-associated lymphoid tissue, most commonly arise in the stomach. MALT lymphomas that arise in the stomach because of *H. pylori* are generally treated successfully with antibiotics that eliminate the bacteria.

Sarcoma and Gastrointestinal Stromal Tumors (GIST)

Sarcomas are a group of cancers that occur in connective tissue, bones, and muscle. GIST is a type of new classification of benign and malignant tumors that include sarcomas that can arise anywhere along the gastrointestinal tract. About 40 to 70 percent of GISTs arise from the stomach, 20 to 40 percent from the small intestine, and 5 to 15 percent from the colon and rectum. About half of these tumors are found in the stomach, yet they are the least prevalent malignant tumors of the stomach. The most common manifestation of gastric sarcoma is upper GI bleeding because of an ulcer forming in the gastric muscosa overlying the tumor. Abdominal pain, anorexia, nausea, vomiting, weight loss, and feeling full are all symptoms. Sometimes these tumors are found incidentally, as they are in Japan, where there is mass screening for gastric cancer with upper endoscopy. There is no standard treatment for malignant gastric stromal tumors, and chemotherapy or radiation seems to have no advantage over doing nothing at all. In 2002 the FDA approved Gleevec (imatinib mesylate) for GIST. Surgery is the treatment of choice and offers the only chance for cure. The tumor is removed with clear margins of at least two centimeters.

Carcinoid

A gastrointestinal carcinoid, or gastric carcinoid tumor, is rare and has some risk of malignancy. Multiple gastric carcinoid tumors are associated with hyperplasia, chronic atrophic gastritis, and pernicious anemia. Type I gastric carcinoids are small, benign tumors associated with gastritis. Type II may be large and prone to spread to the lymph nodes. Type III gastric carcinoids are large, solitary, sporadic tumors that are not associated with any particular gastric condition. They tend to metastasize to the lymph nodes and liver.

Other Disorders of the Stomach

Sword swallowers probably injured their stomachs quite often, but most people are unlikely to suffer this type of injury. Stomach injuries are usually caused by accidents or surgery. And other than swords, people have been known to swallow small objects that get stuck in their stomach, such as dentures and pins. A more common disorder is gastroparesis, which causes food to remain in the stomach.

Gastroparesis

Diabetics often develop gastroparesis, a disorder in which the stomach doesn't empty properly. The movement of food is controlled by the vagus nerve. If it is damaged, the stomach and intestinal muscles don't operate normally, and this slows the passage of food. The vagus nerve in a diabetic is damaged when glucose levels are too high for too long. Glucose causes chemical changes in the nerves and also damages the blood vessels that carry oxygen and nutrients to the nerves. The disorder affects the pacemaker of the stomach. Sometimes it weakens the stomach muscle itself so it can't respond to the pacemaker.

What happens to food if it isn't moving? It stays in the stomach, ferments, and hardens into a solid mass, known as a bezoar, which can block the passage of other food and cause nausea and vomiting. Bacteria can overgrow the fermenting food.

When food that has been delayed in the stomach does finally enter the small intestine, it is absorbed, but blood glucose levels rise. This makes blood glucose levels erratic and difficult to control and is a serious complication for a diabetic.

While diabetes is the main cause of gastroperesis, other causes include:

- smooth muscle disorders such as amyloidosis and scleroderm
- nervous system diseases such as Parkinson's and abdominal migraine
- metabolic disorders, including hypothyroidism
- postviral syndromes
- anorexia nervosa
- surgery on the stomach or vagus nerve

Scars and fibrous tissue from ulcers and tumors can block the stomach outlet and mimic gastroparesis. Certain drugs weaken the stomach, such as tricyclic antidepressants such as Elavil, calcium blockers such as Cardizem and Procardia, L-dopa, and narcotics. Reflux disease can cause it, too, but this is rare. In many cases the cause of gastroparesis is unknown.

Symptoms of Gastroparesis

Symptoms depend on the cause, but these are some:

- heartburn
- nausea
- vomiting of undigested food
- feeling full after eating even small amounts
- weight loss
- abdominal bloating
- erratic blood glucose levels
- loss of appetite
- reflux
- spasms of the stomach wall

Diagnosis of Gastroparesis

Diagnosis begins with the medical history to look for symptoms. If gastroperesis is caused by anything other than diabetes, an upper endoscopy and ultrasound may be called for. The endoscopy would reveal any abnormalities in the stomach lining. The ultrasound would rule out problems in the gallbladder and pancreas. These tests can confirm a diagnosis of gastroparesis.

Barium X-ray

This requires a twelve-hour fast that under normal conditions would result in an empty stomach. After drinking barium to coat the inside of the stomach, an X-ray is taken. If it shows food still in the stomach, gastroparesis is likely. However, if the test shows an empty stomach, you may have to repeat the test. With gastroparesis, sometimes food is digested and sometimes it is not, so the test could be false. Naturally, diabetics need to follow doctors' orders carefully when fasting.

Barium Beefsteak Meal

For this test, the barium is mixed into your food before the pictures are taken. The radiologist will be able to watch the stomach as the meal is digested and see how long it takes. This shows how well—or not—the stomach is digesting food. Emptying problems that don't show up on the barium X-ray may show up on this test.

Radioisotope Gastric-Emptying Scan

For this test, food such as scrambled eggs is mixed with a radioisotope, that is slightly radioactive but not dangerous. After eating, you lie under a machine that follows the food with the isotope as it goes through the stomach. If more than half the food remains in the stomach after two hours, gastroparesis is suspected.

Gastric Manometry

This measures the electrical and muscular action in the stomach. A thin tube is passed down the throat into the stomach. The tube contains a wire to take the measurements as food and liquid are digested.

Upper Endoscopy

This should be done to be sure there is no blockage in the stomach.

Electrogastrogram (EGG)

This measures the electrical waves that normally sweep over the stomach and precede each contraction.

Blood Tests

These measure chemical and electrolyte levels.

See chapters 2 and 3 for more information about these tests.

Treating Gastroparesis

When diabetes is the cause of gastroparesis, treatment is focused on controlling the blood glucose levels with insulin, oral medications, and diet changes. Any underlying cause of the disorder needs to be treated first. When gastroparesis is severe, intravenous or tube feeding may be necessary. In most cases the gastroparesis won't be cured, but it can be kept under control.

Medications

Reglan (metoclopramide) stimulates stomach muscle contractions. This helps empty the stomach and reduce nausea and vomiting. It is usually taken before meals and at bedtime. Side effects include fatigue and sometimes anxiety or depression. There also may be problems with physical movement. Erythromycin is an antibiotic that improves stomach emptying by increasing the contractions that move the food. Abdominal cramps and nausea are side effects. Motilium (domperidone) has been used in other countries with some success. However, it has not been approved by the FDA and its importation into the United States was curtailed when it was discovered that some women who breastfeed were using the drug from foreign sources to increase breast milk production. Domperidone may increase the secretion of prolactin, a hormone that is needed for lactation. Propulsid (cisapride) is used for severe nighttime heartburn in adults with reflux disease that does not respond to other therapies. It is no longer marketed in the United States because it was associated with heart-rhythm abnormalities. However, patients with debilitating conditions for whom the benefits outweigh the risks can ask their doctors to contact the drug company, which will make the drug available as part of a limited access protocol. Other medications may be used to help relieve the nausea and vomiting. Antibiotics are used to clear up infections. If there is a bezoar, it can be dissolved by injecting it with medication through an endoscope.

Diet

Diet and nutrition must be addressed. Eating six small meals a day rather than three large ones is one way doctors advise patients to deal with gastroparesis. This may put less pressure on the stomach, and it can do its work more easily. Some doctors recommend several liquid meals a day until the blood glucose levels are stable. These meals can provide all the needed nutrients and pass through the stomach more quickly. Avoidance of high-fat and high-fiber foods also may be prescribed. Fat takes longer to digest than other foods, and fiber also is difficult to digest. In fact, some high-fiber foods such as cabbage or broccoli contain material that is not digested. The undigested food can form into a bezoar.

Feeding Tube

If medications and dietary changes don't work, then a feeding tube needs to be inserted surgically. The tube is called a jejunostomy tube and goes through the skin of the abdomen into the small intestine. This is a useful and temporary therapy when the gastroparesis prevents medications and nutrients from getting into the bloodstream.

Parenteral Nutrition

Nutrients can be delivered directly into the bloodstream by bypassing the digestive system altogether. A thin catheter is placed into a chest vein, and a bag is attached. This delivers the liquid nutrients and medications. This, too, is usually a temporary method during a period of difficulty with the gastroparesis. It is used only when other methods don't work.

Other Treatment Methods

A gastric neurostimulator is a battery-operated pacemaker surgically implanted in the stomach. It gives off mild electrical pulses that stimulate the stomach muscles to contract so food can be digested and moved into the intestines. The electrical stimulation also helps control nausea and vomiting.

The botulinum toxin (botox) can improve stomach emptying and gastroparesis symptoms. Botox is injected directly into the sphincter and decreases the prolonged contractions of the muscle between the stomach and the pyloric sphincter, which opens to let food into the small intestine.

Foreign Bodies in the Stomach

In the previous section, we talked about food or other objects getting stuck in the esophagus and the need to remove them. If such objects get into the stomach, they usually have a good chance of passing all the way through the digestive tract. But this is not always the case. There are at least fifteen hundred deaths a year in the United States because of ingesting a foreign body that may have gotten impacted in the ileocaval valve, where the small and large bowel connect, or the anus. Objects can get stuck in strictures or diverticula. Children, elderly denture wearers, mental patients, and prisoners have a history of ingesting foreign bodies.

Symptoms of Foreign Bodies in the Stomach

Foreign bodies in the stomach don't always result in symptoms. Large ones may cause getting full quickly, vomiting, difficulty eating, or even cause weight loss. Years could go by before somebody has symptoms unless the item is toxic or has perforated an organ.

Diagnosis of and Treating Foreign Bodies in the Stomach

Abdominal X-ray usually will reveal the presence of a foreign body such as a chicken bone or a safety pin. However, even if nothing shows up in the X-ray, an endoscopic examination should be done.

Dr. Patrick G. Brady, professor of medicine at the University of South Florida College of Medicine and chief of the digestive disease section of Haley Veterans Affairs Medical Center in Tampa, has studied this problem extensively. The decision to remove the object depends on what and where it is. Sharp, pointed, and elongated objects such as toothpicks, open safety pins, nails, toothbrushes, and elongated wires should always be removed because the risk of perforation is as high as 35 percent. Long and narrow objects such as wires are dangerous because they won't pass the fixed curves of the duodenum. They can become impacted or perforate the stomach. If the object is blunt or rounded and less than 2.5 centimeters in diameter, it can be watched for two weeks with X-rays. The average time, according to Brady's experience, for a foreign object to transverse the gastrointestinal tract is seven days. Observation should be extended for delays of six days in the duodenum, ten days in the small bowel, or for the development of any complications.

Tiny button or disc batteries are the most frequent type of foreign body ingested. These unsealed batteries have an alkaline content that is toxic when in contact with the mucous membranes. To prevent potential corrosive injury they have to be removed. However, if the battery has cleared the esophagus, it will usually get through the rest of the digestive tract quickly and without difficulty and won't need to be removed unless signs of injury are present.

Endoscopic Removal

Endoscopic tools include accessories for removing foreign bodies from the esophagus and stomach. Surgery is indicated only if the object has caused complications. Before performing endoscopy, however, the object should be duplicated outside of the body and a dry run attempted to determine the best method for extraction.

Functional Stomach Complaints

Quite often people come in to their doctor with gastrointestinal complaints that can't be explained by their primary care physicians. These functional upper GI complaints account for a third to half of referrals to gastroenterologists. Because functional complaints are difficult to understand and treat, the uncertainty often leads to frustration, judgmental attitudes, and ordering inappropriate tests in a futile attempt to find a biological cause. Even when an organic problem is found, it rarely correlates with the symptom or complaint.

Evidence may indicate spasms, delayed gastric emptying, irritable bowel syndrome, or psychological illness. Functional or nonspecific symptoms also may occur, along with a medical disease such as an ulcer, but psychological or cultural factors may more strongly contribute to the presentation of symptoms, making diagnosis difficult and medical treatment insufficient.

Chapter 6
The Small Intestine

THE SMALL INTESTINE is a long, narrow, muscular tube that lies coiled in your abdominal cavity. This is your food processing plant, where nutrients are digested and absorbed. This long route through the small intestine allows time for various enzymes to process proteins into amino acids, carbohydrates into simple sugar, and fat into glycerol and fatty acid.

The duodenum, the shortest part of the tube, is connected to the stomach and receives secretions from the liver, gallbladder, and pancreas. The jejunum and ileum are both long and coiled, but the jejunum is slightly thicker, redder, and shorter than the ileum, which connects to the large intestine.

This tube has four layers, with the innermost layer being the mucosa, which has millions of projections called villi, which increase the surface area and the mucosa's ability to absorb nutrients. Thus the inner lining looks like a hairbrush. Each villus contains a lymph vessel and a network of minute blood vessels and cells that secrete mucus. So, on its trip through the small intestine, everything you eat becomes processed for pickup by the villi for delivery to the bloodstream. Damage to the villi is what causes most problems in the small intestine.

If you were to flatten out the entire area of the small intestine, conceptually it might be like a doubles tennis court. With disease (resulting in damage), the surface area might decrease to the size of a singles tennis court, a badminton court, or even a Ping-Pong table! Absorption of nutrients would accordingly be impaired.

Conditions covered in this chapter include:

- Celiac disease and sprue
- Short bowel syndrome
- Infections
- Whipple disease

- Bacterial overgrowth syndrome
- Chronic idiopathic pseudo-obstruction
- Diverticulosis of the small intestine
- Mesenteric ischemia
- Benign tumors
- Cancer

Celiac Disease

When your small intestine cannot digest the gluten found in wheat and other grains, you have a condition known as celiac disease, also called sprue, or gluten sensitive enteropathy (GSE). This is an immune-mediated disease that runs in families and is often confused with other gastrointestinal conditions such as lactose intolerance, because symptoms may be similar. Celiac disease also is called nontropical sprue, but it is not the same as tropical sprue, an intestinal infection that affects people living in the tropics.

Celiac disease affects mostly Caucasians of western European heritage while largely ignoring Chinese, Japanese, and people of Afro-Caribbean background. It is the most common genetic disease in Europe, especially England, Ireland, Spain, and Italy. In Italy about 1 in every 250 people has it. In Ireland the tally is slightly lower, with 1 in 300. An estimated 1 in 4,700 Americans has the condition. We don't really know why it is not more prevalent in the United States when so many Americans come from European groups where it is common. It may be that it is underdiagnosed and many people here don't know they have it. Until we have more research, we won't know the true prevalence of celiac disease here. Recent studies show increased prevalence in eastern Europe, South America, and northern Africa.

Celiac disease was first reported in 1888, but it was not until 1950 that wheat was proposed as the cause. The evidence was based on the observation of a Dutch physician named W. K. Dicke, who noted that during World War II, a time when wheat grains were so scarce in Holland, children with celiac disease who had otherwise failed to thrive improved on a wheat-poor diet. Since then the large water-insoluble protein gluten, present in wheat, has been identified as the offending substance. Gluten is a wheat storage protein, and gliadin is the alcohol-soluble fraction of the gluten. Celiac disease is really intolerance to gliadin. A cross-reaction to related rye and barley proteins also causes disease. In 1953 studies with other doctors, Dr. Dicke noted that if wheat is banished from the diet and rice flour, maize starch, or boiled potatoes are given instead, the vomiting and abdominal pain disappear and the patient gains weight and, if not yet an adult, growth in height. By 1954 Dr. Dicke identified the histologic damage to the intestinal mucosa.

When you have celiac disease you have an immune reaction to gluten, which is found in wheat, rye, barley, and possibly oats. When you eat these foods your immune system responds by attacking and damaging the small intestine. This is more like an immune system–mediated inflammation reaction than a classical allergy. The tiny fingerlike protrusions called villi on the lining of your small intestine absorb nutrients from food and send them into the bloodstream. Without villi to carry out absorption you become malnourished—regardless of how much food you eat.

While celiac disease is initiated by an immune mechanism, there is a familial component because it runs in families. There is a 10 percent prevalence of the disease in first-degree relatives—grandparent, parent, sibling—of someone with the disease. This doesn't mean that those relatives will get it, however.

The disease is associated with certain HLA genes that are in charge of the body's immune system. In someone with celiac disease, the genes tell the intestinal system to attack the gliadin protein, and in the process, the small intestine becomes damaged and inflamed. As a result there is decreased absorption. Fewer than 5 percent of people with celiac disease have an immune enteropathy that is not specific for gliadin.

When celiac disease leads to malnutrition, weakness, iron deficiency, anemia, and neurological problems such as peripheral neuropathy, a tingling numbness in the legs can occur. Failure to absorb enough calcium can lead to osteoporosis. For the disease to be properly diagnosed the doctor needs a high index of suspicion.

Symptoms of Celiac Disease

Not everyone is affected the same way by celiac disease. Some people develop symptoms as children, while others don't have them until well into their adult years. Children with this disease usually have symptoms by the time they are two years old, and 20 percent of cases occur in people over sixty. The disease may remain dormant for years and be triggered—or become active for the first time—by pregnancy, childbirth, surgery, a viral infection, or severe emotional stress.

Breast-feeding is thought to play some role in when and how celiac disease appears. If you were breast-fed, symptoms may develop later in life. Another factor may be the age when you began eating foods containing gluten and how much of these foods you ate.

For unknown reasons, the three classic symptoms of celiac disease—diarrhea (often nocturnal), weight loss, and abdominal pain—are rarely observed today. Symptoms may or may not occur in the digestive system. One person may have diarrhea and abdominal pain, while another has irritability or depression. This irritability is one of the most common symptoms of the disease in children.

A thirty-two-year-old woman suffered from intermittent diarrhea, gaseousness, and bloating for several years. At times she noted "oil" in the toilet with her stools as well as undigested food. And despite a healthy appetite, she had recently lost weight and was anemic. A small-bowel series X-ray revealed an abnormal pattern to the small intestinal mucosa. An endoscopic biopsy of the small intestine showed profound inflammation. Once she was on a gluten-free diet, her symptoms went away. Follow-up endoscopy showed that the lining of her small intestine had returned to normal.

When no symptoms are present, it could mean that the undamaged part of your small intestine is able to absorb enough of the nutrients to prevent symptoms. Even without symptoms, the condition will progress and lead to malnutrition or other conditions.

Diagnosis of Celiac Disease

In the past, correctly diagnosing celiac disease was sometimes delayed because symptoms were similar to those of irritable bowel syndrome, Crohn's disease, diverticulosis, intestinal infections, ulcerative colitis, and even chronic fatigue syndrome. The good news is that recent research has revealed that people with celiac disease have higher than normal levels of certain antibodies in their blood. The immune system produces antibodies in response to substances it perceives as a threat, such as bacteria.

IgA is an antibody produced in the mucous membranes of the nose, throat, lungs, and gut. The body produces IgA in response to foreign substances (antigens) that are breathed in or ingested with food. Within the immune system there is a genetically based sensitivity to gluten, so when you eat it, your body makes IgA. To diagnose for celiac disease, your doctor will measure levels of these antibodies to gluten: antigliadin, antiendomysium, and antireticulin. If you have celiac disease, you have specific antibodies. These can be determined using a tube of blood sent to the appropriate laboratory.

In addition to a blood test, your doctor will want a biopsy of the small intestine for a definitive diagnosis. This can be done with an endoscope, a long, thin tube inserted through your mouth and into your small intestine. This instrument can see the lining and also snip off a piece that can be viewed under a microscope. Characteristic intestinal changes usually occur during childhood, but in many cases, diagnosis is not made until years later, as adults. Under the microscope, the tissue from inside the small intestine looks flattened, indicating that the villi are not erect and doing their job. Diagnosis can only be confirmed, however, if a later biopsy shows a change as a result of a gluten-free diet. Lack of response to a gluten-free diet (with a positive blood test) is called refractory sprue (see below).

Your doctor also needs to rule out other conditions with similar symptoms, such as lactose intolerance, Whipple's disease, infections, and other gastrointestinal and autoimmune conditions.

Treating Celiac Disease

Ninety percent of people with celiac disease are cured once they go on a gluten-free diet. This stops symptoms, heals existing intestinal damage, and prevents further damage. Improvements begin within days of beginning the diet, and in three to six months the intestinal damage is healed. For older adults this may take longer, sometimes up to two years.

Omitting gluten can seem as if you are being deprived of your favorite foods and beverages, but today there are many tasty and easily available alternatives. Once you get into the swing of this diet, you will not feel deprived. Gluten-free breads, pasta, and other products are available in health food stores and via the Internet. Many commercial food stores also carry gluten-free foods.

Although you may easily adapt to your diet at home, you need to be especially cautious when eating in restaurants, school cafeterias, and at cocktail parties, where you cannot be sure of ingredients. Gluten is often used in preservatives, additives and stabilizers in processed foods, medicines, and even mouthwash. Most processed foods such as salad dressings, frozen and packaged meals, desserts, and soups contain gluten-based preservatives or stabilizers. When ingredients are not listed on a label, avoid the product until you can contact the manufacturer and find out what's in it.

You need to avoid anything with these ingredients:

- wheat (gliadin); also spelt, triticale, and kamut
- rye (secalin)
- barley (hordein)
- oats (avenin); these are well tolerated once healing is well under way

It is mandatory that your doctor refer you to a dietician who can help you learn more.

A Guide to Gluten-Free Substitutes

Here are just a few examples of foods you can substitute:

- *Alcoholic beverages.* You cannot have beer or malt or grain whiskey . . . but you can have sake, plum wine, or tequila.
- *Bread, cereal, pasta.* You cannot have graham crackers, wheat or rye bread, or oatmeal . . . but you can have rice, hominy grits, quinoa flakes, puffed rice, and breads made with potato, corn, soy, or other flour.
- *Soups, salad dressings, seasonings.* You cannot have creamed soups, prepared gravies, salad dressings, and even some brands of ketchup or chili or curry mixes, but you can have clear broth, homemade soups, and salad dressings.
- *Desserts.* You cannot have Krispy Kremes, Dunkin' Donuts, or most bakery products, but you can have all of those things prepared with substitute ingredients.

There also are support groups you can find on the Web and through your health-care system. These groups often have information about gluten-free diets and commercial products that are gluten-free—or not. They are:

American Celiac Society: amerceliacsoc@netscape.net

Celiac Disease Foundation: www.celiac.org and cdf@celiac.org

Celiac Sprue Association/USA: www.csaceliacs.org

Gluten Intolerance Group of North America: www.gluten.net and info@gluten.net

American Dietetic Association: www.eatright.org and hotline@ eatright.org

Gluten-Free Living (newsletter): gfliving@aol.com

You can find a database for gluten-free food on the Internet at www.nowheat.com. Other Web sites of interest are:

www.glutensolutions.com

www.authenticfoods.com

www.glutenfree.com

A Diet for Life

Once your symptoms go away, you may be tempted to reintroduce foods containing gluten to see the response. What harm to put your pastrami on rye bread? Don't do it. At first you may feel no symptoms, but they will gradually reappear after a period of latency. In some cases the symptoms come back with greater force and it will be more difficult to control them. You may then need medications in addition to the diet.

A thirty-year-old lawyer, who was progressing nicely on his gluten-free diet, had a relapse over pizza. This was the one thing he most missed. Occasionally he would stop for a slice, enjoy it, and feel guilty. When it became apparent after a few months that his gluten-free diet wasn't working as well as it should, he finally confessed to his pizza problem. He was encouraged to try to make his own pizza with gluten-free flour. Granted, homemade pizza may not be as authentic and satisfying, but it is a valid substitute, and once you learn how to make it, can be quickly accomplished.

Will You Need Vitamin Supplements?

Talk with your doctor about adding vitamin supplements to your diet. Depending on how long you've had celiac disease, you may be deficient in some vitamins. For example, breads, cereals, and other wheat products contain important B vitamins. Folic acid or folate is needed for regeneration of cells, and almost all celiac patients are deficient in this vitamin. If deficiencies in other nutrients such as iron, calcium, or magnesium were present before diagnosis, you may need supplements.

When Diet Is Not Enough: Refractory Sprue

A very small number of people with celiac disease may not improve on the gluten-free diet. They may have severely damaged intestines that won't heal even when gluten is removed from their diets. This often happens in older people who may have had the disease for a long time. Their bodies need help in reducing inflammation. Some may need to receive intravenous nutrition supplements, but this is rare. Regeneration of villi occurs quicker in children, but regrowth/healing should be accomplished by one year in most celiacs of all ages.

Diagnosis of Refractory Sprue

About 75 percent of people with refractory sprue have abnormal mono-clonal T cell outgrowth. Expression of monoclonal T cell populations is a risk factor for developing overt lymphoma. This means they may also be a risk factor for nonlymphoma. Thus chronic refractory sprue may be a precancerous condition.

Treating Refractory Sprue

About 10 percent of people with refractory sprue will require immuno-suppressive therapy with medication. Glucocorticoids such as oral pred-nisone usually are given first. Other medications include azathioprine (Imuran) and cyclosporin. There are drug treatments being researched now that may be even more effective.

Screening for Early Diagnosis of Celiac Disease

Most Americans are not routinely screened for antibodies to gluten. However, if you have first-degree relatives with this disease— grandparent, parent, sibling—then tell your doctor to have you tested. And if you have the disease, advise your other relatives to get tested. The longer the condition is untreated, the greater your chance of developing the condition.

Because the disease is common in Italy, all children there are screened for celiac disease by age six so it can be caught early, even if no symptoms are present. Italians of any age also are tested as soon as they show symp-toms. This vigilance by the Italian health-care system means that the time between when symptoms occur and the disease is diagnosed is usu-ally two or three weeks. In the United States, however, the time between symptoms and diagnosis is about ten years.

Complications and Associated Conditions

Because unchecked celiac disease damages the small intestine, the result-ing malabsorption puts you at risk for malnutrition, osteoporosis, miscar-riage, and even neurological complications. Other conditions associated with celiac disease are type 1 diabetes, autoimmune thyroid disease, microscopic colitis, rheumatoid arthritis, Down syndrome, peripheral neuropathy, and Sjögren's syndrome. Having these and more associated conditions means more people should be screened.

Non-Hodgkin's Lymphoma

You have a greater risk of getting non-Hodgkin's lymphoma (NHL), a cancer of the lymphatic system, if you have celiac disease. In fact, small intestinal NHL occurs at a rate sixteen to fifty times higher with celiac disease than without it. Lymph nodes are in various parts of the body, including the villi of the small intestine. Lymphocytes are the cells in this system, and malignant lymphocytes—B and T cells—are involved in this type of cancer. B cells produce antibodies, and T cells direct the traffic in the immune response system. However, early dietary management of celiac disease and reduced symptoms reduce this risk.

Dermatitis Herpetiformis

In some people gluten intolerance can cause a severe itchy, blistering skin disease called dermatitis herpetiformis (DH). A rash usually develops on the elbows, knees, and buttocks, but it also can appear on the scalp, neck, shoulder, and lower back. Lesions first appear as discolorations and then small bumps called papules and small blisters called vesicles. They tend to appear in groups, much like the lesions of herpes, from which it gets its name meaning, "like herpes."

Although DH is related to celiac disease, since both are immune disorders, they are separate diseases. People with DH usually have no digestive symptoms, although they often have the same intestinal damage as those with celiac disease. The immunologic findings and changes in the villi are identical with those found in celiac disease. Damage to the intestinal villi occurs in more than 66 percent of patients. DH is often referred to as "celiac disease of the skin."

Typically, DH begins either in the teenage years or in the thirties and forties. There are about one in a million cases in the United States, and men get it twice as often as women. The ethnic differences are the same as for celiac disease—it's common among Europeans and uncommon among Asians and African Americans.

Diagnosis of Dermatitis Herpetiformis

This is done with a skin biopsy. A tiny piece of skin near the rash is removed and tested for the IgA antibody. The only difference between ordinary celiac disease and DH is where the IgA antibodies go. In celiac disease, the gastrointestinal tract is the main target organ. In DH the main targets are the epithelial cells—the skin.

Treating Dermatitis Herpetiformis

This involves oral medication for the rash and a gluten-free diet to prevent further disease. Dapsone or sulfapyridine may provide rapid relief of the itching in a day or two, but drug treatment may last several years. Glucocorticoids may be used in severe disease. On a gluten-free diet and without drugs, it takes about two years for the rash to disappear.

As there may be various side effects to the drugs, the gluten-free diet is the better route. Many people tend to think that if the drug works, why bother with the diet? However, the diet treats the cause rather than the symptoms.

During and after treatment you would need to be monitored with monthly blood tests to check for anemia.

Chronic Fatigue Syndrome

People with chronic fatigue syndrome may be more vulnerable to celiac disease according to some medical studies. This direction began when similar blood serum markers were present in patients with both conditions. Some investigators are looking into the possibility that undiagnosed celiac disease might be the cause of diverse clinical symptoms, especially in patients who are tired all the time.

Tropical Sprue

Tropical sprue is not hereditary, like celiac disease (nontropical sprue), but the symptoms are similar. It is a digestive problem that occurs in the tropics and subtropics. The cause has not been identified, but it probably is an infection by a microorganism. As in celiac disease, the villi, the fingerlike projections in the lining of the small intestine, are attacked by the disease and fail to function, thus making absorption of nutrients difficult.

Tropical sprue affects about one in a million people near the equator. It is more common in India, Haiti, Cuba, Puerto Rico, and the Dominican Republic, but rare or absent in Africa, the Bahamas, and Jamaica. Residents as well as travelers who stay for a month or more can contract the disease.

Symptoms and Diagnosis of Tropical Sprue

Symptoms are similar to those of nontropical sprue, but other factors are involved such as nutritional deficiency and a transmissible infection, or toxin. It even may begin months or years after you have returned from the tropics. Diarrhea is the main symptom, and this is more severe if you eat lots of fatty foods. Other symptoms include cramps, weight loss, gas, and indigestion.

Diagnosis can be complicated because symptoms are similar to those of any number of gastrointestinal problems. Blood and stool tests have to be done to rule out other causes of the diarrhea. If you have been living in the tropics for a month or more and there is no other diagnosis, you probably have tropical sprue.

Because the disease causes lack of absorption of certain vitamins and minerals, blood tests may need to be done to be sure you do not become malnourished. You may have low levels of albumin, calcium, or vitamin D. You also may have anemia due to vitamin B_{12} and folate deficiencies. There may be excessive amounts of fat in your stool, because it could not be absorbed properly. Malabsorption of at least two nutrients is required for diagnosis. A jejunal biopsy is not very specific, but usually it shows shortened and thickened villi.

Treating Tropical Sprue

Treatment with antibiotics leaves most people symptom-free within weeks. Two to four weeks of sulfonamide or doxycycline therapy usually gets good results. Supplements of folic acid and vitamin B_{12} may be added to the treatment. Most people are cured forever, but about 20 percent may have a recurrence after treatment.

The only way to prevent the disease is to avoid staying in tropical climates for prolonged periods.

Other Disorders of the Small Intestine

Although celiac disease is the most common disease of the small intestine, that organ is susceptible to any number of infections as well as short-bowel syndrome and cancer.

Short-Bowel Syndrome

This condition occurs when the functions of the small bowel have been removed by disease or surgery. Crohn's disease in the form or regional enteritis (inflammation) is the most common cause of short-bowel syndrome (SBS). As you know, the small intestine is more than twenty feet long and divided into three sections. First is the duodenum, a short section about a foot long, just beneath the stomach. Next is the jejunum, the largest but not the longest section. The final three-fifths of the small intestine is the ileum, which connects to the large intestine.

The difficulty of living with a shortened small intestine depends on which sections are affected. Half of the small bowel can be removed without causing too much disability, especially if the ileum is not involved. But the more intestine removed, the greater the disability. The entire jejunum can be removed and the ileum will compensate, but lactose intolerance may result. If the ileum is removed, more problems will occur because it is responsible for absorption of fats, bile salts, and vitamin B_{12}.

Although Crohn's disease is the most common cause of SBS, there are others. Surgical removal of the ileum because of a volvulus (twisted bowel) is one. Severe traumatic injury or any surgery that causes the ileum to be bypassed also can induce SBS.

The symptoms of SBS depend on how much of the small bowel is lost and how long the resulting malabsorption has continued. In general there is weight loss, diarrhea, bloating, fatigue, and steatorrhea (fat in the stool). If malabsorption is long-standing, there may be anemia and other signs of nutrient deficiency. All symptoms occur because the body cannot absorb nutrients such as fats, carbohydrates, electrolytes, vitamins, and minerals.

Rachel, thirty, developed severe abdominal pain during the eighth month of her second pregnancy and was rushed to the hospital. Preliminary tests revealed blockage in her small intestine because part of it was twisted. Rachel underwent a C-section to deliver the baby safely, and then several feet of small intestine had to be removed to bypass the twisted area. Initially treated with parenteral nutrition, Rachel is now home maintaining her weight and eating a diet rich in supplements and vitamins. She has had some episodes of partial small intestinal obstruction but has not needed further surgery.

Treating Short-Bowel Syndrome

There are three stages of medical management of SBS: total parenteral nutrition (TPN), oral feedings, and total adaptation. TPN provides nutrition intravenously. It begins slowly and increases gradually to avoid causing diarrhea and high blood sugar. Then it is slowly stopped and a transition is made to a basic oral diet of foods that are easy to digest. This is done through a nasal feeding tube. Gradually more complex foods are added until the patient is weaned off the infusions. Once back on regular eating, the patient must be monitored by a physician to avoid any complications.

Transplantation

Sometimes medical treatment doesn't work and a transplant is required. According to the United Network for Organ Sharing, about 670 intestinal transplants have been performed in the United States since 1990. More patients probably would get them if there were more awareness. Transplantation of the small bowel has among the highest success rates among transplantations.

Infections of the Small Intestine

A variety of infections can take up residence in the small intestine. Some are self-limiting, but others become chronic for years. Most infections will interfere with the work of the small intestine, which is to digest, absorb, and propel food through the gut. As a result, diarrhea is a common symptom. Others include bleeding, bloating, nausea, vomiting, abdominal pain, and sometimes obstruction. Here are some of the infections:

Campylobacter Infections

This is a very common cause of diarrhea in the United States affecting over a million people a year. It is caused by handling raw poultry or eating it undercooked. (One drop of juice from a raw chicken can infect you.) Failure to wash cutting boards and utensils used for raw poultry, and then using them for other foods, is how it spreads to other foods and then to you. When a large outbreak occurs, it is usually because of drinking unpasteurized milk or contaminated water. (Men are more prone to this than women.) Most people recover in two to five days without any specific treatment. However, in severe cases, antibiotics are used.

Salmonella

There are many types of salmonella, but the most common is food poisoning. The organism is common in meat products, with chickens and eggs probably the most common causes of infection. Symptoms usually begin within ten to forty-eight hours after eating contaminated food and can range from mild gastroenteritis to severe diarrheal illness with dehydration. If you have other diseases, such as sickle-cell anemia or heart valve disease, you may be at risk for a more profound form of the disease that disseminates through the blood. Most people get better spontaneously, but if they are ill, antibiotics are used.

Typhoid Fever

This is from a particular species of salmonella. It produces prolonged fever, bacteria in the blood, and multiple organ dysfunctions, including inflammation of the kidney and brain. Typhoid fever is rare in the United States, and immunization can prevent it. Treatment is with powerful antibiotics and specific therapy if other organs are involved.

Staphylococcus aureus

This is probably the second most common cause of bacterial food poisoning in the United States. It occurs when food is prepared by people who are infected with strains of the staphylococcus but show no symptoms. The bacteria multiply in food and produce the toxin, which is not killed by heating. Symptoms of vomiting and cramping develop in six to eight hours, but recovery is usually within twenty-four to forty-eight hours.

Bacillus cereus

This is an organism that causes food poisoning. It is associated with cooked foods such as fried rice that are kept out too long without refrigeration, especially foods in restaurants. Vomiting usually occurs within six hours of eating the food, and some people develop diarrhea. Most improve without treatment.

Protozoal Infections

These include Giardia lamblia and come from parasites that contaminate water supplies and often occur in travelers in underdeveloped countries. Children in day-care centers and the adults working with them also have a higher incidence of contracting this type of infection. Symptoms vary but include gaseousness, bloating, and sometimes weight loss. Diagnosis usually is made with specific stool analysis or with upper endoscopic biopsy. Antibiotics are used to treat this type of infection.

Intestinal Worms

These are common around the world including the United States. Tapeworms attach themselves to the lining of the small intestine and are the most common cause of iron deficiency anemia worldwide. This also can result in stomach pain and diarrhea. There are several varieties of tapeworms. Some are found in fish, beef, and pork and infection is transmitted from poorly cooked meats. The most common tapeworm in the United States is thought to be transmitted through contact with human feces. Tapeworms can obstruct the intestine but usually cause few symptoms apart from occasional diarrhea and abdominal pain. The fish tapeworm can cause vitamin B_{12} deficiency. Other worms, such as strongyloides stercoralis and echinococcus, are less common in humans in the United States.

Other Infections

Other infections that can cause symptoms include various *E. coli*, clostridium, shigella, yersinia, and vibrio (cholera). There are also viral infections of the intestine that can bring on diarrhea and dehydration.

Whipple's Disease

Whipple's disease is a systemic disease most likely caused by bacteria (*Tropheryma whippelii*), that causes malabsorption in the small intestine, and also affects the joints, central nervous system, and cardiovascular system. It is so rare, however, that fewer than five hundred cases have been reported in medical literature. It is also fatal after one year if it is not correctly diagnosed and treated. Middle-aged men are the most common targets of this disease.

Whipple's disease usually presents as a classic wasting illness with arthritis, fever, and diarrhea. Swollen lymph glands also may occur. If the disease affects the small intestine, steatorrhea (fatty liver) often is present. Weight loss, occult bleeding, and diarrhea are symptoms. Swelling of the joints also may occur.

Whipple's disease is treated with antibiotics.

Bacterial Overgrowth Syndrome

The small intestine was once believed to be a sterile environment, with the bacteria needed for assisting digestion firmly rooted in the large intestine. This is not always the case. Bacterial overgrowth occurs when the normally low bacterial colonization in the upper gastrointestinal tract increases significantly. This can occur with low gastric acidity, reduced peristalsis, or damage to the mucous lining. Although very rare, this syndrome can cause wasting or failure to thrive and prolonged diarrhea. No particular bacteria have been implicated, but abnormally large numbers of them are the cause.

In the United States, about 20 to 40 percent of chronic diarrhea patients with diabetes are associated with bacterial overgrowth syndrome. In many cases, gastric and upper GI surgery is the cause. It is the cause of about half the cases of neonatal chronic diarrhea. These babies as well as the elderly are at highest risk.

Breath tests can diagnose the condition, which can be treated with antibiotics aimed at restoring the balance of bacterial flora. Treatment also is aimed at reducing the damage caused by malabsorption and restoring nutritional health and normal gut flora. Without prompt treatment, malnutrition can occur.

Small-Bowel Obstruction

The leading cause of small-bowel obstruction in industrialized countries is postoperative adhesions followed by malignancy, Crohn's disease, and hernias, although some studies have reported Crohn's disease as a greater factor than cancer. Surgeries most closely associated with this condition are appendectomy, colorectal surgery, and gynecologic and upper gastrointestinal procedures. In this country, small-bowel obstruction accounts for 20 percent of hospital admissions for abdominal complaints. The obstruction can be partial or complete, simple or strangulated. A strangulated obstruction is a surgical emergency because if it is not treated it can lead to loss of blood supply and death.

Symptoms include crampy, intermittent abdominal pain. This is usually followed by nausea and vomiting. Diarrhea may occur early in the episode and constipation later as evidence that bowel contents are not passing all the way through the tract. Fever and tachycardia may occur late. The condition can be diagnosed with abdominal X-rays and CT scan. Antibiotics must be administered, followed by surgical treatment to remove the obstruction.

Chronic Idiopathic Intestinal Pseudo-obstruction and Ogilvie's Syndrome

Chronic idiopathic intestinal pseudo-obstruction (CHIP) and Ogilvie's syndrome are similar rare conditions characterized by recurrent episodes of symptoms and signs of intestinal obstruction—but without any evidence of a mechanical obstruction. There is no organic explanation and no apparent cause. CHIP can be acute or chronic and affect the small or large intestine. Ogilvie's syndrome affects the colon. When seen on radiographic tests, both conditions reveal what looks like a bowel obstruction. If the colon is affected, it may become massively dilated and this presents a risk of perforation, peritonitis, and death. Symptoms include abdominal pain, nausea and vomiting, constipation, and fever.

More than thirteen thousand orthopedic and burn patients have been documented with this obstruction, but the true incidence of it remains unknown because it resolves spontaneously. It generally develops in hospitalized patients and is associated with a variety of medical and surgical conditions such as trauma; severe infections; and cardiothoracic, pelvic, or orthopedic surgery. Pregnancy and cesarean delivery also have been the cause. Certain medications, such as narcotics, anticholinergics, clonidine, amphetamines, phenothiaszines, and steroids, also have been implicated.

Blood tests, liver function profile, and testing of electrolytes are required for proper diagnosis. Plain X-rays and CT scans can identify symptoms and rule out other possible causes of the symptoms, such as perforation.

Medical care includes treating any underlying condition, administering fluids to correct electrolyte imbalance, and discontinuing any medications that may be part of the problem. If the problem is in the small intestine, a cecostomy may be needed. This is generally open surgery, but laparoscopic surgery can be done. In rare cases, surgery may be necessary for colonic venting.

Diverticulosis of the Small Intestine

Although diverticulosis is quite common in the large intestine, it is rare in the small intestine. A diverticulum is a small, saclike herniation of the intestine that protrudes outside through weak points in the intestinal wall. Why it develops in the small intestine is unknown, but it may result in abnormal peristalsis. Other possible causes include a low-fiber, high-fat diet, advancing age, or systemic sclerosis. In the United States duodenal diverticula are approximately five times more common than jejunoileal diverticula. The actual incidence of both types is unknown because they rarely cause any symptoms and usually are discovered at autopsy. When symptoms develop they include abdominal pain, anemia, bleeding, and diverticulitis accompanied by fever and local tenderness.

Diagnosis can be made with X-rays or CT scan and treatment may include antibiotics and possibly surgery (see chapter 3).

Mesenteric Ischemia

When the flow of blood to all or part of the small intestine occurs, mesenteric ischemia develops. The condition is related to heart disease such as cardiac arrhythmias, recent myocardial infarction, and congestive heart failure. It usually happens to older people. Shock also can be a cause. Symptoms include abdominal pain, sometimes related to meals. Nausea, vomiting, and diarrhea are frequent. Surgery is required to remove the blockage. Untreated, this condition leads to gangrene and death.

There are chronic and acute forms of mesenteric ischemia. Half of the acute cases are due to artery occlusion from an embolism. A quarter of cases are due to an infarction. The rest are due to inferior artery occlusion.

Benign Tumors of the Small Intestine

Benign tumors of the small intestine are so rare that they often cause no symptoms and are discovered only during autopsies. These tumors may develop alone or in groups of several types, such as hyperplastic polyps, adenomas, GI stromal tumors, and hemangiomas. They grow slowly in any part of the small intestine and may be part of a polyposis syndrome. These tumors are so rare because intestinal transit through the small bowel is swift, so there is little time for the bowel contents to remain in contact with the bowel lining. Also, the contents at this phase of digestion contain more fluid than later, when they get to the colon. The alkaline pH also may play a role in keeping the bacteria count low.

Cancer of the Small Intestine

Cancer of the small intestine is very rare. You are fifty times more likely to get cancer in your colon than in your small intestine. Doctors in this country diagnose about twelve hundred malignant tumors of the small intestine a year, a small number compared with the frequency of tumors elsewhere in the digestive tract. The liquid nature of the contents of the small intestine and the speed of transit through the long length of it may reduce exposure of cancer-inducing agents to the intestinal wall. Other protective factors may be a low bacterial count, a high alkaline pH environment, a large lymphoid tissue component in the wall of the small bowel, and the presence of the enzyme benzpyrene hydroxylase.

There are two types of cancer that affect the small intestine. The most common type is adenocarcinoma, which begins in the lining of the small intestine. Tumors occur most often in the upper part of the small intestine, close to the stomach. These often grow and block the passageway. Other types are sarcoma and carcinoids. Leiomyosarcomas, even less common, grow in the smooth muscle lining of the small intestine.

Adenocarcinomas occur most often in industrialized countries, while lymphomas are more common in developing countries. When adenocarcinoma does occur in the small intestine it usually is associated with Crohn's disease, celiac disease, or familial polyposis syndromes. All of these tumors can invade the intestinal wall, spread into adjoining lymph nodes, and metastasize to distant organs.

Symptoms include pain or cramps in the middle of the abdomen, unexplained weight loss, a lump in the abdomen, or blood in the stool. Diagnosis is usually done with an upper GI series, a CT scan, MRI, or ultrasound. A biopsy will be done via upper endoscopy.

Treatment for cancer in the small intestine is with surgery, radiation, chemotherapy, or a combination of these therapies. Specific treatment depends on the stage of the cancer. The part of the intestine with the cancer can be surgically removed and reconnected to the healthy parts. If the doctor believes all of the cancer was removed with surgery, he or she may add chemotherapy treatment to be sure all cancer cells are killed. Radiation therapy can be internal or external. Clinical trials are ongoing using biological therapy, which tries to get the body's own immune system to fight the cancer.

Chapter 7
The Gallbladder

THE GALLBLADDER is a pear-shaped sac that hangs like a little pod from a tree branch. This pod and its branch—the cystic duct—are attached to the common hepatic duct, which comes from the liver. These ducts lead into the common bile duct, which is attached to the duodenum, the entry to the small intestine. All the ducts from the liver and the gallbladder itself form the biliary system, often called the biliary tree for obvious reasons.

The liver produces bile, a yellow-green liquid that helps digest fats and rid the body of certain waste products. Bile is made of water, lecithin, cholesterol, bile salts, and bilirubin. It is carried through bile ducts from the liver into the gallbladder, where it is stored and concentrated. When you eat fat-containing foods your gallbladder contracts and ejects the bile back through the ducts and into the small intestine, where it helps digest the fat.

If the liquid bile contains the wrong proportion of cholesterol, bile salts, or bilirubin, under certain conditions it can harden into stones that can block or interfere with the normal flow of bile. The result can be a sharp pain or a painful spasm on the right side, or in the midline of the upper abdomen just under the rib cage. Sometimes you can feel the pain radiate to your back under the right shoulder blade. Symptoms often flare after meals (especially high-fat meals) because the gallbladder normally contracts after you eat fatty, greasy, or oily foods.

When a stone blocks the outflow of bile, the gallbladder becomes inflamed, a condition called cholecystitis. Gallbladder inflammation without stones present, called acalculous cholecystitis, may be brought on by prolonged fasting, severe illness, or for no obvious reason. Cancer can develop in the gallbladder and the biliary ducts, but this is rare. In this chapter, you'll find out what to do about:

- Gallstones
- Cholecystitis
- Acalculous cholecystitis
- Biliary dyskinesia
- Cancer of the gallbladder and biliary tree

Gallstones

Most of the twenty million Americans who have gallstones never notice them. Even if the stones are discovered by a doctor, in most cases there's no need to treat them unless they begin to cause discomfort and pain. Treatment usually consists of surgically removing the gallbladder. The body works just fine without a gallbladder, and digestion proceeds normally.

There are two main types of gallstones: cholesterol stones and pigmented stones. In America, most people have the cholesterol gallstones; in Asia, gallstones are more often pigmented. Gallstones can be as small as a grain of sand or as large as a golf ball. The gallbladder can develop just one large stone, hundreds of tiny stones, or almost any combination. It is believed that the mere presence of gallstones may cause more gallstones to develop. Small gallstones may exhibit mobility, while large stones often sit tight.

Cholesterol Stones   These are usually yellow-green and are made primarily of hardened cholesterol. Scientists believe that cholesterol stones form when bile contains too much cholesterol, too much bilirubin, or not enough bile salts (a fat-dissolving detergent), or when the gallbladder does not empty as it should for some other reason. More than 75 percent of these stones are found in people living in developed countries. Larger stones are associated with cholecystitis. Smaller ones can travel down the digestive system to where the ducts join the pancreas. These are associated with pancreatitis.

Pigment Stones   These are small, black or brown stones made of bile pigment—bilirubin—combined with calcium. They tend to develop in people who have cirrhosis of the liver, biliary tract infections, or hereditary blood disorders such as sickle-cell anemia, in which too much bilirubin forms. Old red blood cells when removed from the bloodstream by the spleen release the red-pigmented hemoglobin. Hemoglobin is converted to the yellow-pigmented bilirubin, which is then excreted by the liver and released into the bile. If the body destroys too many red cells (a condition called hemolysis), excess bilirubin is produced and thus pigment stones can form in the gallbladder. Sickle-cell anemia causes early destruction of red cells, and many people with this condition have a gallbladder operation by age twenty.

Calcification of Stones   This frequently occurs, resulting in their becoming hardened. About 15 percent of stones contain so much calcium that they can be seen on plain X-rays as calcified, or hardened. Calcification of cholesterol stones typically occurs only at the rim. Calcified gallstones may be resistant to efforts to dissolve them.

Biliary Sludge   This is thickened gallbladder mucoprotein with tiny cholesterol crystals that may be a precursor of gallstones. Typically this sludge causes biliary pain, cholecystitis (acalculous), or acute pancreatitis. It is often found during pregnancy, during prolonged intravenous feeding, rapid weight loss, or starvation.

The Risk of Getting Gallstones

If you are an overweight, middle-aged women or a Native American man or woman, you are at the highest risk of having gallstones. Twice as many women as men get gallstones, and all people over sixty are more likely to develop gallstones than younger people. Up to 10 percent of all adults in the West have them. The following factors can predispose one to having gallstones:

- *Obesity.* This is a major risk factor, especially in women. A number of clinical studies showed that being even moderately overweight increases your risk for developing gallstones. The risk is especially high in people with the highest body mass index. Obesity tends to reduce the amount of bile salts in bile, resulting in more cholesterol, and it also decreases gallbladder emptying.
- *Rapid weight loss.* As the body metabolizes fat during rapid weight loss, it causes the liver to secrete extra cholesterol into bile, which can cause gallstones. There is some controversy over whether conventional dieting to lose weight causes gallstones.

- *Fasting.* Prolonged starvation decreases gallbladder movement, causing the bile to become overconcentrated with cholesterol, which can lead to gallstones. People who are receiving long-term intravenous feeding face this risk.

- *Elevated estrogen production.* Pregnancy, hormone replacement therapy, or birth control pills appear to increase cholesterol levels in bile and decrease gallbladder movement, both of which can lead to gallstones. Estrogen decreases bile acid production, thus decreasing the solubilization of cholesterol.

- *Ethnicity.* Native Americans have a genetic predisposition to secrete high levels of cholesterol in bile. In fact, they have the highest rate of gallstones in the United States. Among the Pima Indians of Arizona, 70 percent of women have gallstones by age thirty. A majority of Native American men have gallstones by sixty. Mexican American men and women of all ages also have high rates of gallstones. Some studies have indicated that Scandinavian women may be at a slightly higher risk than other women.

- *Cholesterol-lowering drugs.* Drugs that lower cholesterol levels in the blood actually increase the amount of cholesterol secreted in the bile. This in turn can increase the risk of gallstones.

- *Low caffeine intake.* Apparently coffee—with caffeine—stimulates gallbladder contraction and thus lowers the risk of gallstones in women.

- *Sedentary lifestyle.* This puts you at a 30 to 40 percent increased risk compared to people who engage in recreational physical activity. In other words, physically active people have 30 to 40 percent fewer cholecystectomies, surgery to remove the gallbladder.

- *High triglyceride levels.* Your total cholesterol level is not a risk factor for gallstones, but elevated fatty acids called triglycerides are clearly linked to gallstone formation. A low level of HDL cholesterol also may be associated with gallstone disease. HDL is the good cholesterol, as opposed to LDL, which is unhealthy. People with diabetes generally have high levels of triglycerides.

- *High red blood cell turnover.* People with anemia, sickle-cell disease, thalassemia, hereditary spherocytosis, elliptocytosis, or liver dysfunction (jaundice) are at higher risk.

Symptoms of Gallstones

Gallstones don't always cause problems. "Silent stones" are sometimes discovered during diagnostic tests for other problems but don't interfere with gallbladder, liver, or pancreas functions. Some people feel pain after eating fatty foods but have no other symptoms. When gallstone symptoms occur, they may do so suddenly, and for that reason are often called a gallstone attack. Typical symptoms of gallstones include:

- Nonspecific abdominal pain
- Steady pain to the right upper abdomen that increases rapidly and lasts from thirty minutes to several hours
- Pain in the back between the shoulder blades or under the right shoulder
- Nausea and vomiting
- Abdominal bloating, belching, and gas
- Recurring intolerance of fatty foods
- Colic
- Indigestion

When severe, symptoms are similar to those of heart attack, reflux disease, appendicitis, ulcers, irritable bowel syndrome, hiatal hernia, pancreatitis, and hepatitis. Accurate diagnosis is critical.

More urgent symptoms   Gallstones can become a more serious problem if they acutely block bile ducts. If you have any of the following, see a doctor right away because your condition could be more serious, such as gallbladder infection or itching (pruritis), a frequent complication of cholestasis, the stoppage of bile flow. Symptoms of pancreatitis also could cause a severe knifelike pain in the back.

- Sweating
- Chills
- Low-grade fever
- Yellowish color of the skin or whites of the eyes
- Clay-colored stools

Diagnosis of Gallstones

Ultrasound is the most sensitive and specific test for gallstones. It detects 85 to 90 percent of stones; provides good visualization of the ducts and thickness of the gallbladder wall; and will reveal cholecystitis, an infection of the gallbladder. When a technician glides a handheld device over your abdomen, he or she is bouncing sound waves off your gallbladder. Their echoes make electrical impulses that create a picture of the organ on a video monitor. The sound waves will reveal the location of stones.

Sometimes additional tests are needed if there is a suspected infection or other complications:

- *Endoscopic ultrasonography.* This is even more precise than external ultrasound. An endoscope can be inserted into your digestive tract to send sound waves and images back directly from the site.

- *Cholescintigraphy (HIDA) scan.* This is used to diagnose abnormal contraction of the gallbladder or an obstruction when ultrasound doesn't provide enough visualization, such as in cases of acute cholecystitis. Overall, it may be the most sensitive test for acute cholecystitis. It also works with people who have had prior gallbladder surgery or poor gallbladder emptying, and those who have eaten just before the test.

- *Computerized tomographic (CT) scan.* While only able to visualize about half of the gallstones, this provides good visualization of the entire liver and pancreas to spot any complications.

- *Endoscopic retrograde cholangiopancreatography (ERCP).* This is used to evaluate (and possibly treat) common bile duct stones. Magnetic resonance cholangiopancreatography (MRCP) uses MRI to visualize the gallbladder, biliary tree, pancreas, and pancreatic ducts.

- *Laparoscopic common bile duct exploration.* This is well tolerated and as safe as ERCP. This is an extension of laparoscopic cholecystectomy, laparosocopic removal of the gallbladder.

Refer to chapter 3 for more information about these tests.

Treating Gallstones

If you have gallstones that don't bother you, you would do nothing, except perhaps to take steps to reduce the risk of making the condition worse by being overweight or sedentary.

Surgery

Each year more than five hundred thousand Americans have a cholecystectomy—surgery to remove their gallbladder. It's the most common way to treat symptomatic gallstones. Anyone with gallstones that cause pain and other symptoms is a candidate for surgery. Someone with chronic anemia or sickle-cell disease or other conditions of the blood and liver also should have their gallbladders removed. So should children with gallstones. If you are at high risk for gallbladder cancer (see page 136), you should have surgery sooner rather than later.

You can live perfectly well without your gallbladder. Once it is removed, bile flows out of the liver through the ducts and goes directly into the small intestine instead of being stored in the gallbladder. However, because the bile isn't stored in the gallbladder, it flows into the small intestine more frequently, causing diarrhea in about 1 percent of people.

Most cholecystectomies are done with laparoscopic techniques. Because the abdominal muscles are not cut during laparoscopic surgery, there is less pain and fewer complications than after open abdominal surgery. Recovery usually involves only one night in the hospital, followed by several days of restricted activity at home.

The surgeon inserts surgical instruments and a miniature video camera right into the abdomen through several tiny incisions. The camera sends a magnified image from inside the body to a video monitor, providing a close-up view of the organs and tissues. While watching the monitor, the surgeon uses the instruments to carefully separate the gallbladder from the liver, ducts, and other structures. Then the cystic duct is cut and the gallbladder removed through one of the small incisions. If the surgeon discovers any obstacles to the laparoscopic procedure, such as infection or scarring from other operations, the operating team may switch to open surgery. In some cases the obstacles are known before surgery and open surgery is planned.

Open abdominal surgery is used in about 5 percent of cases because the gallbladder is infected, or because other complications have developed. A five-to-eight-inch incision is made across the abdomen to remove the gallbladder. This is a major surgery and may require two to seven days in the hospital and several more weeks of recovery at home.

The most common complication to gallbladder surgery is injury to the bile ducts. If the common bile duct is injured, it can leak bile into the body and cause a painful and potentially dangerous infection. Mild injuries sometimes can be treated, but a major injury usually requires additional surgery. Follow the advice of your surgeon with regard to diet, activity, and follow-up care.

Endoscopic Retrograde Cholangiopancreatography

If gallstones are in the bile ducts, they can be located and removed with endoscopic retrograde cholangiopancreatography (ERCP) before or during gallbladder surgery. In ERCP you literally swallow an endoscope—a long, flexible, lighted tube connected to a computer and a TV monitor. The doctor guides the endoscope through your stomach and into the small intestine, where a special dye is injected to temporarily illuminate the biliary ducts. When the affected duct is located, an instrument on the endoscope cuts the duct. The stone is captured in a tiny basket and removed with the endoscope.

A high school principal, James was fifty-three and healthy until he began to experience upper abdominal pain, malaise, mild jaundice, dark urine, and pale stools. A test showed he had elevated liver enzymes, but he did not have hepatitis. A sonogram revealed gallstones and a dilated common duct. He was referred to a gastroenterologist and underwent an ERCP with papillotomy. The procedure improved drainage of bile from the biliary tree into the duodenum, and four small stones were swept from the common bile duct. However, he elected to have his gallbladder removed via laparoscopic cholecystectomy to prevent any possible future problems.

Occasionally a gallstone in a duct is diagnosed weeks, months, or even years after the cholecystectomy. The two-step ERCP procedure is usually successful in removing the stone.

Dissolving the Stones

Some gallstones can be dissolved medically, leaving the gallbladder intact. If you have small, uncalcified stones and a functioning gallbladder, your doctor may prescribe dissolving stones with ursodiol (Actigall). This is a bile salt that helps dissolve the cholesterol in bile. Cholesterol crystals are dissolved from the outside to the inside. It's not effective, however, with large stones or calcified pigment stones and is relatively slow-acting. Ursodiol is taken two or three times a day depending on your body weight, and continued for several months after the stones no longer appear on ultrasound. After six months, about 37 percent of stones dissolve. This process needs to be watched via ultrasound every six to twelve months, or years of treatment may be necessary before all the stones dissolve. It may cause mild diarrhea. The drug does not work for everyone and stones could re-form once the drug is stopped.

Ursodiol therapy is effective if you have infrequent attacks and small gallstones, or if surgery would be risky for you. It also is used as a preventive for anyone in a rapid-weight-loss program. But you must have stones that have not calcified, and the cystic duct must allow the dissolving agent to enter the gallbladder. It is used as a maintenance therapy in elderly and high-risk surgical patients.

Diane, sixty-five, was in poor health from chronic cardiac and respiratory conditions. She had upper abdominal discomfort after meals and was found to have many small noncalcified cholesterol gallstones, but her gallbladder was functioning. Because she was a poor operative risk, she was treated with a low-fat diet and ursodiol. After two years a sonogram showed no gallstones present.

Lithotripsy—shock waves that crush stones—sometimes may be used for small stones. The procedure is more commonly used for kidney stones.

What about Diet?

Although diet cannot dissolve gallstones, it may help reduce the frequency and severity of painful attacks. Lose weight if you need to, and follow a low-fat diet. Eating less fat, for example, puts less demand on the gallbladder, so it contracts less forcefully. Dietary fiber reduces the amount of cholesterol in the bile, and the tendency to form gallstones also is reduced. By changing the chemical composition of the bile through diet, it is possible to halt the growth of stones, or in rare cases even cause the stones to shrink.

If you are trying to lower triglycerides, be sure to avoid sweets and to control the amount of carbohydrates you eat (starchy foods such as pasta, bread, and potatoes).

Other Conditions of the Gallbladder

Several conditions of the gallbladder, from infection to cancer, cause symptoms that are often difficult to diagnose because they are so similar to other digestive diseases.

Acute Cholecystitis

A sixty-year-old overweight woman had complained to her primary care physician for months about pain in her abdomen and in her back. She had been under treatment for other problems, and the doctor dismissed her complaints as psychosomatic. One evening after a heavy dinner, she had pain in her upper abdomen and back so acute that she thought she was having a heart attack. Her family rushed her to the hospital, where it was discovered that her gallbladder was so badly infected, gangrene had already set in. She was admitted to the hospital, and her gallbladder was removed. This woman's gallstones had been ignored for so long, her gallbladder could have become perforated at any moment. She had acute cholecystitis—or infected gallbladder. Cholecystitis, or infection of the gallbladder, most often occurs in the setting of gallstones.

Symptoms and Diagnosis of Acute Cholecystitis

Symptoms are the classic triad of right upper abdominal pain, elevated white blood cells (leukocytosis), and fever. Pain is so acute it can lead to a change in mental status. When the cystic duct is blocked, the gallbladder becomes distended. It can't function and shuts down. There is vascular compromise as well, with decreased blood flow to the gallbladder. A cystic duct obstruction is usually caused by a gallstone. Bacterial overgrowth occurs and may lead to infection, especially in older people. It is often called ascending cholangitis when the infection proceeds to the common bile duct. About 45 percent of people with blocked ducts will develop secondary bacterial infections in other sites of the body.

Careful diagnosis is crucial here, and doctors must rule out peptic ulcer disease, acute pancreatitis, right lower lobe pneumonia, hepatitis, nephrolithiasis, appendicitis, or adhesions due to pelvic inflammatory disease (PID), all of which may share some of the symptoms.

Treating Acute Cholecystitis

Once the bacteria have been identified, antibiotics are prescribed to control the infection. However, normal eating must cease, and intravenous fluids are used for hydration while the antibiotics work. If doctors can stabilize your condition, they may delay surgery for twenty-four to forty-eight hours to make you a better operative candidate.

Surgery to remove the gallbladder is standard, but ERCP-based therapies may be used to enlarge the common bile duct to allow a large stone to be extracted if it is lodged in the common bile duct. Enlargement is accomplished by sphincterotomy and papillotomy, transection of the biliary sphincter, a valve that regulates the flow of bile and pancreatic juices into the duodenum. Electrocoagulation is usually used, and the result is a sphincterectomy, or removal of the valve, which is effective in 85 percent of cases.

Common bile duct exploration with a laparoscope (a surgical procedure done at the time of a laparoscopic cholecystectomy) is as safe and effective as ERCP.

Acalculous Cholecystitis

Acalculous cholecystitis is a clinical condition characterized by pain in the biliary ducts without the gallstones. We don't know what causes it, but it is probably due to an abnormal gallbladder motility that may cause a relative obstruction of the cystic duct. This condition seems to occur in women more than men, but we don't know how many people have it. Pain usually develops in the right upper quadrant thirty to sixty minutes after meals and lasts from one to four hours. It is often exacerbated by greasy and spicy foods. Nausea is common, but vomiting is unusual.

Several hormones affect the motility of the gallbladder, and because women are more often victims of this condition, female sex hormones are suspected of playing a role. An ultrasound usually can find the condition.

Patients frequently undergo extensive, often invasive and expensive, testing before they get definitive therapy. There is no effective medical care, and the condition usually is treated surgically with laparoscopic cholecystectomy or intraoperative cholangiography. Surgeons tend to label acalculous cholecystitis as biliary dyskinesia (see below). But to gastroenterologists, biliary dyskinesia is a synonym for sphincter of Oddi dysfunction, which is a distinct disease process.

Biliary Dyskinesia

Biliary dyskinesia is defined as biliary colic without the gallstones, but the diagnosis and treatment are controversial. A severe, steady pain occurs in the upper right quadrant of the abdomen and lasts for thirty minutes or more. The pain is steady, interrupts daily activity, and leads to a doctor visit. There is no evidence of structural abnormalities, but the gallbladder is not emptying properly.

An ultrasound examination can rule out gallstones or lesions. If gallbladder emptying is normal, ERCP should be considered as treatment. Also, if the gallbladder is emptying, it could be a dysfunction of the sphincter of Oddi. In addition, pain may be associated with elevated liver or pancreatic enzymes and/or conjugated bilirubin. Biliary dyskinesia may be associated with acute pancreatitis. Treatment options include medication or sphincterotomy.

Cancer of the Gallbladder or Bile Ducts

Cancer of the gallbladder or bile ducts is not common, but women get it more often than men, and it is more common in people who have gallstones. Symptoms are similar to gallstone problems, and in the early stages there may be no symptoms at all. Most of the cancers are discovered because of symptoms such as jaundice, abdominal pain, unexplained weight loss, or discovery of the "porcelain gallbladder" when radiography is done for some other reason.

A gallbladder is considered porcelain when there is extensive calcium encrustation. The term emphasizes the blue discoloration and brittle consistency of the gallbladder wall at surgery. We don't know how many people have such gallbladders, but the male-to-female ratio is one to five. Ninety percent of porcelain gallbladders are associated with gallstones. Often people have no symptoms, and porcelain is found accidentally during X-rays or other diagnostic testing. When it is diagnosed, however, the porcelain gallbladder should be removed because of the high risk (22 percent) of cancer.

All the standard diagnostic tests for gallbladder problems may fail to uncover cancer, and it is often found during open abdominal surgery, when the surgeon can visualize the internal organs and examine them. By then the cancer has usually metastasized.

Primary cancer of the gallbladder is a highly fatal disease that will afflict more than six thousand adults in the United States every year. Typically it is not discovered until it is well advanced, so it is difficult to remove it all during gallbladder surgery.

The cause has eluded scientists so far, but it has been associated with gallstone disease, estrogens, cigarette smoking, obesity, alcohol consumption, and being female. The incidence of cancer involving the biliary tract is ten times higher in patients with ulcerative colitis and Crohn's ileocolitis. The tumor usually sprouts in the neck of the gallbladder, then spreads along the wall and directly into the liver. If it goes in the opposite direction, it spreads into the small bowel and pelvis. When diagnosed, most of the gallbladder has already been destroyed by the cancer, and about half the patients have regional lymph node metastases.

In the United States, the highest incidence is in New Mexico, where there is a large population of Native Americans and Mexicans. Worldwide, Israel has the highest incidence, followed by Mexico, Bolivia, Chile, and northern Japan. Low rates are found in India, Nigeria, and Singapore. Gallbladder cancer is most often diagnosed in people in their sixties.

Risk Factors for Gallbladder Cancer

The primary risk factors for gallbladder cancer are having long-term gallstones, particularly symptomatic and large ones, or cholecystitis. If you have what is known as a "porcelain gallbladder," you are at risk for this cancer.

Gallbladder polyps, while not uncommon, may in some cases add to your risk of cancer. Most of these polyps do not cause cancer. They consist of cholesterol, muscle tissue, or inflammatory tissue. Some polyps, however, are adenomatous, and this type can progress to cancer. The risk is related to the size of the polyp—the larger it is, the greater the risk. Most polyps are discovered as incidental findings at the time of gallbladder sonography.

Being overweight also is a risk factor.

Cholangiocarcinoma is cancer of the bile ducts, and there are several types of bile duct tumors:

- Type I: tumors below the confluence of the left and right hepatic ducts

- Type II: tumors reaching that confluence

- Type IIIa: tumors occluding the common hepatic duct and the right hepatic duct

- Type IIIb: tumors occluding the common hepatic duct and the left hepatic duct

- Type IV: multicentric (Klatskin) tumors that involve confluence and both hepatic ducts

Risk Factors for Bile Duct Cancer

There are some conditions that put you at higher risk for cancer in the biliary ducts. A bile duct adenoma is one. So are choledochal cysts, which usually are present in childhood; these are more common in Japanese people. Caroli's disease is another risk. This is a rare, congenital condition of cystic dilation of the bile ducts. Having multiple biliary papillomatosis, a tumor that blocks the ducts, also is a risk factor.

If you have sclerosing cholangitis, your lifetime risk of getting bile duct cancer is 10 to 30 percent. This is a condition where the bile ducts inside and outside the liver become inflamed and scarred. As the scarring increases, the ducts become blocked. Ulcerative cholitis also puts you at risk, even without sclerosing cholangitis.

In other countries this cancer can be caused by various parasites that affect the biliary tree.

Smoking also is regarded as a risk factor. It should be noted, however, that most cases of cholangiocarcinoma occur in patients without risk factors.

Diagnosis of Gallbladder or Bile Duct Cancer

A CT scan or a CT-guided needle biopsy are the recommended diagnostic tests for gallbladder cancer. Magnetic resonance imaging (MRI) is more sensitive, gives additional information, and is likely to replace CT for initial assessment. Endoscopic ultrasonography can be used to visualize the farther reaches of the biliary tree. Cholangiography is the most important method for assessing whether the tumor should be removed surgically. Once cancer is found, it can be assessed—or staged—to indicate the best treatment. The stages are as follows:

- Stage 0: carcinoma in situ. This means the cancer is contained within the gallbladder or the duct
- Stage I: tumor invasion is limited to mucosa, muscle layer, or ampulla
- Stage II: tumor has spread to local area
- Stage III: cancer has spread to regional lymph nodes or adjacent tissue
- Stage IV: extensive invasion of liver or adjacent structures/organs, distant metastasis

Treating Cancer of the Gallbladder or Bile Ducts

Once cancer is found, more tests will be done to determine if it has spread. If the cancer is contained within the gallbladder, it can be removed completely. If it has spread to the liver, stomach, pancreas, or intestine or lymph nodes, other treatments may be more appropriate.

Part of the liver around the gallbladder and some lymph nodes in the abdomen also may be removed just in case any cancer cells have moved into those areas. Laparoscopic cholecystectomy is effective for Stage 0 and Stage I gallbladder cancers.

If the cancer has spread, surgery also may be done to relieve symptoms. For example, if the tumor has blocked the bile ducts, and bile is building up in the gallbladder, a biliary bypass can be done surgically to relieve this. The gallbladder or bile duct can be cut and sewed to the small intestine. When ducts are removed, biliary stents, or artificial ducts, can replace them. Palliative surgery also appears to improve survival with bile duct stent placement.

With surgery or other procedures, a catheter can be installed to drain the bile that has built up in the area. The drain can go directly into the small intestine, or it can come outside the body.

Anyone with cirrhosis of the liver or major cardiopulmonary disease would not be a candidate for surgery.

Radiation or chemotherapy may be added to treatment after surgery, but these tumors are resistant to chemotherapy and radiation.

Survival rates for cancers in the gallbladder or biliary ducts are low: about 5 percent of patients live five years. However, clinical trials always are in progress, and new treatments are being developed. For information call the Cancer Information Service at 1-800-4-CANCER (1-800-422-6237). TTY at 1-800-332-8615.

Chapter 8

The Pancreas

THE PANCREAS is a large, solid gland shaped like a fish with a head, body, and tail. It is about the size of a human hand and sits behind the stomach, close to the duodenum, the upper part of the small intestine. It is larger than the gallbladder and smaller than the liver, both of which are nearby. The gland is divided into two distinct sections. The endocrine section produces insulin, which it secretes into the bloodstream along with glucagon, somatostatin, and pancreatic polypeptide. The exocrine section secretes digestive enzymes into the small intestine through a tube called the pancreatic duct. These enzymes help digest fats, proteins, and carbohydrates in the food we eat. The exocrine section also secretes a bicarbonate-rich fluid that helps neutralize stomach acid.

In this chapter you'll find out what to do about:

- Acute and chronic pancreatitis
- Pancreatic cancer

Pancreatitis and Pancreatic Cancer

Normally, digestive enzymes do not become active until they reach the small intestine, where they begin digesting food. But if these enzymes are blocked by gallstones in the duct, or because of some other problem, they become active inside the pancreas. A current theory is that these trapped enzymes start "digesting" the pancreas. In other words, they attack the tissue that is producing the enzymes. The pancreas becomes inflamed, and pancreatitis results. However, this theory is not yet proven. If it were, then high-dose drugs to inhibit enzyme production would work—but they don't.

Very high levels of inflammatory proteins are observed in people with pancreatitis, and emerging evidence suggests that lack of oxygen (ischemia reperfusion) plays a central role. There is accumulating evidence that oxidant stress resulting from an excess of pro-oxidant over antioxidant has a key role. From this it would seem likely that therapy with antioxidants should help to prevent pancreatitis, especially recurrent pancreatitis. Some studies have shown this to be true, and antioxidant therapy is under investigation in clinical trials.

Acute pancreatitis comes on suddenly, lasts for a short period of time, then goes away. Chronic pancreatitis does not resolve itself and results in the slow destruction of the pancreas. Either form of pancreatitis, when severe, can cause serious complications such as bleeding, tissue damage, and infection. Fluid-filled sacs of tissue—pseudocysts— also may develop. Enzymes and toxins can get into the bloodstream and injure the heart, lungs, kidneys, or other organs.

The risk of pancreatitis for African Americans between thirty-five and sixty-four is ten times higher than for whites or any other group. In the United States, Native Americans have the lowest rate. Men and women are equally at risk.

Acute Pancreatitis

It's possible to have more than one attack and recover completely after each one, but acute pancreatitis also can be a severe, life-threatening illness with many complications. About 20 percent of the eighty thousand cases that occur in the United States each year are severe.

More than half of cases of acute pancreatitis are caused by gallstone obstruction of the pancreatic duct. Small stones, about the size of a pencil eraser, and mulberry-shaped stones are the major risk factors. A gallstone can block the pancreatic duct, trapping digestive enzymes in the pancreas rather than letting them go into the small intestine and do their work. A buildup of biliary sludge—coagulated digestive enzymes—also can cause an attack. Alcoholism can be blamed for at least 20 percent of cases; high triglyceride levels (more than 500mg/dL) account for another 15 to 20 percent. Certain prescription drugs also can lead to pancreatitis. Drugs known to induce acute pancreatitis include:

- Diuretics: thiazides, furosemide, ethacrynic acid, and chlorthalidone
- Immunosuppressive drug azathioprine
- Antibiotics: sulfonamides, tetracycline, rifampicin, and metronidazole
- Antiepilepsy drug sodium valproate

- Corticosteroids and the anti-inflammatory drug indomethacin
- Estrogens in birth control pills and hormone replacement therapy
- Diabetes drug phenformin
- Antidiarrheal drug diphenoxylate
- Stomach acid-lowering drug cimetidine

Pancreatic or intestinal abnormalities or tumors, abdominal trauma, or damage from an endoscopic procedure also can cause pancreatitis. In rare cases the disease may result from viral infections such as mumps or cocksackie virus infection, and people in western states have been known to develop pancreatitis from scorpion stings, but this is rare. In about 15 percent of cases the cause is unknown.

Linda, twenty-nine, went to a hospital emergency room with severe pain in her upper abdomen and mild midabdominal pains hours after eating a large restaurant meal. Blood tests and a CT scan confirmed the diagnosis of pancreatitis. Further evaluation with endoscopic retrograde cholangiopancreatography (ERCP) revealed that Linda had pancreas divisum, a congenital abnormality where a double duct system drains the pancreas. This has been associated with acute, recurrent, and chronic pancreatitis.

Hereditary Pancreatitis

Hereditary pancreatitis (HP) is a rare disorder, characterized by recurrent episodes of pancreatitis, often beginning in early childhood. Although some of the genes involved have been identified, there is a complex pattern involved in the inheritance, and we believe that other genes are involved.

Less than 1 percent of all pancreatitis is hereditary because of mutations in the cationic trypsinogen gene (PRSS1). If two or more family members have pancreatitis in more than one generation, then it is probably hereditary. The condition begins when a child is ten to eleven years old and leads to frequent acute attacks and ultimately to chronic pancreatitis. Although the disease is generally mild and some people with genetic mutations have no symptoms, they are at a fifty-three times greater risk for pancreatic cancer. It's not clear that everyone with a family history of the disease should get genetic testing because there still is no way to prevent the disease.

Symptoms of Acute Pancreatitis

Acute pancreatitis usually begins with knifelike pain in the upper abdomen (epigastrium) that radiates to the back. It may be a steady, burning pain that feels worse when you move or lie down and eases if you sit up and lean forward. It has been described by medical people as one of the worst pains a person can feel. It often makes people look and feel very sick.

Other symptoms include:

- Fever from infection
- Weakness, lethargy, feeling light-headed from low blood pressure
- Nausea, anorexia, vomiting
- Dehydration (can indicate internal bleeding)
- Tachycardia (can indicate shock)

Complications of Acute Pancreatitis

Acute pancreatitis also can cause breathing problems such as hypoxia. Doctors treat this by giving oxygen through a face mask. Despite treatment, some people still experience respiratory failure and require intubation and a ventilator. This may progress to adult respiratory distress syndrome.

The pancreas can hemorrhage, internal infection can occur, an abscess could form, and the cells of the pancreas can die. These are serious conditions that can lead to a medical and surgical emergency and require critical care monitoring. If bleeding occurs in the pancreas, shock and sometimes even death follow. Anyone with sudden onset of severe abdominal pain needs to see a doctor and be evaluated.

Chronic Pancreatitis

With chronic pancreatitis, the gland is abnormal before and/or after an attack. Not only is it swollen and inflamed, but also cell death—necrosis—is nearly always present. The ducts are usually blocked, and tissue has become calcified. This progressive disease slowly destroys the cells of the exocrine pancreas, until it can no longer process the enzymes necessary to digest food. Once the exocrine pancreas is destroyed, the endocrine pancreas also will deteriorate, resulting in diabetes, when more than 90 percent of the gland has been destroyed. Fifteen percent of people with chronic pancreatitis become insulin-dependent. Chronic pancreatitis also doubles the risk of pancreatic cancer. Overall, 4 percent of people with chronic pancreatitis for more than twenty years will develop this cancer.

The inability to digest food results in malabsorption and weight loss. This means that no matter how much you eat, the food is not nourishing you because it is not being digested and absorbed into the bloodstream. People often eat more food because they are never satisfied, but this results in more pain as the diseased pancreas tries to cope.

Chronic disease may cause obstruction of the common bile duct as it passes through the pancreas and secondary biliary cirrhosis. About 15 percent of people with chronic pancreatitis have scarring in the bile duct. Biliary drainage to decompress the duct needs to be done to improve bile flow from the liver. Pancreatic pseudocysts also can develop with chronic disease. They cause no symptoms and usually resolve themselves unless they rupture, hemorrhage, get infected, or block the gastrointestinal tract. In that case they need to be surgically or endoscopically drained. Pancreatic ascites, an accumulation of fluid within the peritoneal cavity, usually occur when cysts or ducts rupture. Fluids also can leak into the pleural space in the chest.

Allison was twenty-eight and had already suffered two attacks of acute pancreatitis. She did not have gallstone, ulcers, or any other risk factor. However, tests revealed a congenital anomaly that results in a double duct system draining the pancreas—pancreas divisum. An attempt was made to correct this condition surgically, but it didn't work. Her pancreatic abdominal pain became even more frequent. From time to time over the years she had oily stools showing partially digested food. Allison was treated with narcotic pain relievers and pancreatic enzyme replacement and was able to function normally.

Alcoholism is the cause of about 70 percent of chronic pancreatitis; but only 5 to 10 percent of heavy drinkers develop the disease. One theory is that the ethanol in the alcohol may increase secretion of insoluble pancreatic proteins that block the ducts. Damage from alcohol abuse may not appear for many years, until a sudden attack of pancreatitis. It is more common in men than in women and often develops between ages thirty and forty.

Children with cystic fibrosis, a progressive, disabling, and incurable lung disease, also may develop chronic pancreatitis. Doctors may overlook this because they focus their attention on the debilitating respiratory problems of patients with cystic fibrosis.

Symptoms of Chronic Pancreatitis

Chronic inflammation of the pancreas causes weight loss because the body does not secrete enough pancreatic enzymes to break down food, so nutrients are not absorbed normally. Fat, protein, and sugar are excreted into the stool, which becomes large and bulky and at times greasy and malodorous.

More than 85 percent of people in this condition have deep midabdominal pain radiating to the back. Sometimes abdominal pain goes away as the condition advances, probably because the pancreas is no longer making digestive enzymes. Often symptoms like those of acute pancreatitis occur, but more frequently.

Diagnosis of Pancreatitis

In addition to taking a medical history and doing a physical exam, a doctor will order blood tests to diagnose pancreatitis. During acute attacks, the blood contains at least three times more amylase and lipase than usual. These are digestive enzymes produced in the pancreas. After the pancreas improves, these levels usually return to normal within seventy-two hours. Lipase is more specific than amylase for pancreatitis. The most impressive increase will occur in a "virgin" pancreas, a gland that has no history of pancreatitis.

With chronic pancreatitis, however, amylase and/or lipase levels may be normal or slightly elevated, as opposed to much higher levels with acute pancreatitis.

Elevated amylase and lipase also may occur with other medical conditions, so doctors must rule out pancreatic or lung cancer, intestinal obstruction, bowel infarction, perforation, renal failure, parotid disease, hepatitis, a ruptured ectopic pregnancy, or macroamylasemia. This last refers to a large amylase molecule that filters very slowly through the kidneys from the blood.

Your doctor also may check for tachycardia and for any reduction in blood pressure. Blood sugar levels and any presence of bilirubinemia are checked as well. In addition, there may be changes in blood levels of calcium, magnesium, sodium, potassium, and bicarbonate. Tests can rule out peptic ulcer, intestinal obstruction, gallbladder disease, kidney and cardiovascular conditions, pneumonia, and diabetic ketoacidosis.

A stool test will detect elevated fecal fat (steatorrhea) due to malabsorption. A liver function test can find abnormalities and deviations that may signify common bile duct obstruction.

In more advanced stages of chronic disease, when diabetes and malabsorption occur, blood, urine, and stool tests help diagnose and monitor the disease.

Imaging Tests

- *Computerized tomography (CT) scan.* This offers the best initial evaluation of the pancreas and is 85 percent specific in chronic pancreatitis.

- *Magnetic resonance cholangiopancreatography (MRCP).* This is a non-invasive method for evaluating the biliary tract, ductal system around the liver, pancreas, and gallbladder. It provides good visualization of ducts with clarity similar to the invasive ERCP. MRCP is especially good for spotting possible tumors in the biliary tree. This test may precede an ERCP in people with low likelihood of intervention.

- *Endoscopic retrograde cholangiopancreatography (ERCP).* This is the gold standard for getting a close look at a pancreas with chronic disease. It is good for seeing the biliary tree, including pancreatic duct(s). Also, gallstones and ductal stones can be removed, and a biopsy can be performed. This is an invasive procedure, but it may be necessary in certain cases.

- *Ultrasound.* This images the gallbladder and liver well but is less sensitive—only 65 percent—with the pancreas.

- *Endoscopic ultrasound.* This technique is increasingly being used to image the fine detail of the pancreas.

- *Plain abdominal X-ray.* This may show pancreatic calcifications in 30 percent of cases, suggesting chronic disease.

- *Angiography.* This is rarely used to view the blood supply in and about the pancreas.

- *Fine needle aspiration.* This is used for evaluating pancreatic masses and cysts.

Refer to chapter 3 for more information about these tests.

Pancreatic Function Tests

When no symptoms show up on the imaging tests but abdominal pain is present, a pancreatic function test is useful although difficult to perform and not readily available. It is about 80 percent sensitive and 85 percent specific.

Pancreatic secretions are collected and tested following a standard meal or an intravenous feeding. A tube is placed through the nose or mouth until its tip is next to the opening of the pancreatic duct. Secretions can be collected and measured. If the bicarbonate and digestive enzyme levels are very low, it can be assumed that the pancreas is not producing sufficiently.

What to Rule Out

Severe pancreatitis is clearly indicated with diagnostic and laboratory findings, but mild or moderate disease may be more difficult to diagnose clearly. In these cases, other conditions need to be ruled out, including:

- Pancreatic cancer (usually painless)
- Peptic ulcer disease
- Irritable bowel syndrome
- Gallstones
- Endometriosis

Treating Pancreatitis

Treatment for acute pancreatitis is designed to relieve pain, support vital functions, and prevent complications. A hospital stay may be necessary so that fluids can be replenished intravenously, to give the pancreas a rest. Any metabolic or nutritional imbalance needs to be corrected.

Painkilling medications such as Demerol are effective, but morphine is not used because it causes sphincter spasm. Somatostatin (Octreotide, Sandostatin), a synthetic form of the hormone somatistatin, inhibits pancreatic secretion and may reduce pain. In some cases, surgery can relieve pain by draining an enlarged pancreatic duct or removing part of the pancreas (see below).

If vomiting cannot be stopped, a tube is placed in the stomach through the nose to remove fluid and air. In mild cases, staying off food for three or four days may help. Fluids, nutrients, and pain relievers can be administered intravenously.

Antibiotics are prescribed for infection, but if it is extensive, surgery may be needed. Surgery also may be used to find the source of bleeding, rule out problems that resemble pancreatitis, or remove severely damaged pancreatic tissue. Antibiotics also are indicated if the pancreas cells are necrotic—dead. However, it's not clear if antibiotics should be used as a prophylactic if there is no evidence of active infection.

If pancreatic pseudocysts are large enough to interfere with the healing of the pancreas, they must be drained radiographically, endoscopically, or surgically.

Unless the pancreatic duct or bile duct is blocked by gallstones, an acute attack usually lasts only a few days. In severe cases, intravenous feeding may be required for three to six weeks while the pancreas slowly heals. This process is called total parenteral nutrition (TPN). However, for mild cases of the disease, TPN offers no benefit.

Removing the Stones

Any stone blocking a duct will have to be removed by enlarging the common bile duct opening to allow the stone to be extracted. This is accomplished through ERCP with sphincterectomy (see chapter 3) and is successful in more than 90 percent of cases. With ERCP the pancreas, pancreatic duct, common bile duct, and/or sphincter of Oddi can be clearly examined. A long, narrow endoscope is passed down the digestive tract to the pancreas to put X-ray dye into the bile and pancreas ducts.

If the pancreatitis is mild, gallstone surgery may proceed within about a week. More severe cases may mean that gallstone surgery is delayed for a month or more. (See chapter 7 about gallstones.) Once the gallstones are removed and inflammation is gone, the pancreas usually returns to normal. ERCP can drain a bile duct that is obstructed due to fibrosis in the head of the pancreas. It's effective in more than 85 percent of cases. In severe cases of pancreatitis, surgery will be needed to drain the pancreatic duct or to remove part of the pancreas.

Pancreatic Enzyme Replacement

Artificial pancreatic enzymes can be taken with meals to improve digestion and lessen pancreatic pain if the pancreas does not secrete enough of its own. The enzymes help the body digest food and correct malabsorption and weight loss. Typical enzyme replacement is six tablets of Viokase four times daily. Acid neutralization with H-2 blocking agents or proton pump inhibitors used to treat heartburn and reflux disease also may be helpful and prevent breakdown of enzyme production. Controlled trials have not yet proven the overall benefit of these treatments.

Platelet activating factor (PAF) antagonist (lexipafant) is showing some promise in treating acute pancreatitis on an experimental basis.

Sometimes insulin or other drugs are needed to control blood glucose in a diabetic patient.

Antioxidant Therapy

High doses of vitamin C and/or other antioxidants may have some benefit, and more studies are under way. Medical researchers in Manchester, England, presented a study in 1998 to the World Congress of Gastroenterology. They used a combination of antioxidant vitamins—beta-carotene, vitamin C, and vitamin E, along with trace minerals selenium and the amino acid methionine—to treat chronic pancreatitis.

These agents are under investigation and should not be used outside of the framework of a clinical trial.

Living with Pancreatitis

Most people with acute pancreatitis have a good future if they take some steps to prevent future attacks. If the cause is gallstones, they will be dealt with surgically.

Obviously, if alcohol is the cause of the condition, then all drinking of alcoholic beverages has to stop. A professional program such as Alcoholics Anonymous and a medical detoxification program are advised, along with a low-fat, high-carbohydrate diet. Here are some other guidelines:

- Get adequate fat-soluble vitamins and calcium in the diet
- Relieve pain with analgesics or surgical nerve block
- Control blood sugar levels by giving insulin
- Take supplemental pancreatic enzymes to correct underproduction

Some Diet Dos and Don'ts

To treat malabsorption, which usually occurs with more than 90 percent destruction of the pancreas, a low-fat diet is desirable.

- Choose lean, protein-rich foods such as skinless chicken, lean meat and fish, soy, and fat-free dairy products.
- Eat foods that are naturally low in fat, such as whole grains, fruits, and vegetables.
- Avoid fried foods, processed foods, and commercially prepared baked goods.
- Limit animal products such as egg yolks, cheeses, whole milk, cream, ice cream, and fatty meats.
- Read food labels and avoid foods with "hydrogenated" or "partially hydrogenated" ingredients. These are loaded with saturated and transfatty acids.
- Olive and other vegetable oil is preferable to butter and margarines made with transfatty acids.

When Your Pancreas Cannot Be Saved

Relief of pain from chronic pancreatitis usually can be achieved only with surgical removal of the pancreas. This is called pancreatectomy, and there is more information on this procedure in the next chapter. The pancreas also is removed to prevent diabetes.

Pancreatic Cancer

Cancer of the pancreas is the fifth-leading cause of cancer death in the United States. About twenty-nine thousand people every year are diagnosed with this cancer, which most often begins in the ducts that carry the pancreatic juices.

We don't know what causes pancreatic cancer, but research has shown that people with certain risk factors are more likely to get it. Having chronic pancreatitis or diabetes are risk factors, as are being over sixty, smoking, being African American, and having a family history of pancreatic cancer.

Because pancreatic cancer doesn't cause any symptoms early in its progression, it is often called a silent disease. As the cancer grows, it produces symptoms such as pain in the upper abdomen and upper back, jaundice, weakness, loss of appetite, nausea and vomiting, and weight loss. These symptoms also are common to other gastrointestinal conditions, so a diagnosis has to be made by ruling out other conditions.

Specific lab tests can be done to check for bilirubin and other enzymes in blood, urine, and stool. Bilirubin passes from the liver to the gallbladder to the intestine. If the common bile duct is blocked by a tumor, the bilirubin cannot pass through, so the levels in the blood, stool, or urine become very high. However, high bilirubin can result from noncancerous conditions, too.

CT scan and ultrasound can view the pancreas. Endoscopic ultrasound as well as ERCP and MRCP may be used to get a more accurate look at the pancreas. (These tests are explained in detail in chapter 3.) A tissue sample can be taken from the pancreas so a biopsy can be done to check for cancer cells. Another way to get tissue for a biopsy is with fine-needle aspiration. Using an X-ray or ultrasound as a guide, the doctor can insert a needle into the pancreas to extract some cells.

Treating Pancreatic Cancer

The treatment will depend on the stage of the cancer, but pancreatic cancer is very difficult to control with current available treatments. Clinical trials often are recommended by doctors who want their patients to get the best possible chance at treatment. Pancreatic cancer can be cured only if it is found at an early state.

Treatment options include surgery, chemotherapy, and/or radiation. Surgery can remove all or part of the pancreas, depending on the location and size of the tumor, the stage of the disease, and the patient's general health.

Whipple Procedure

This can be used if the tumor is in the head or widest part of the pancreas. The head of the pancreas can be removed along with part of the small intestine, bile duct, and stomach. Other nearby tissues also may be removed if cancer may have spread to them.

Distal Pancreatectomy

This is the removal of the body and tail of the pancreas if the tumor is in either of these parts. The spleen also may be removed.

Total Pancreatectomy

This removes the entire pancreas, part of the small intestine, part of the stomach, the common bile duct, the gallbladder, the spleen, and nearby lymph nodes. If the cancer cannot be completely removed and the tumor is blocking the common bile duct, the surgeon can create a bypass to allow fluids to flow through the digestive tract. This can relieve jaundice and pain resulting from the blockage. Sometimes the blockage can be relieved with a stent to avoid surgery. Following surgery, patients are fed intravenously and through feeding tubes into the abdomen. In a few weeks the tubes can be removed and normal eating can resume.

Islet Cell Tumors

A rare form of pancreatic disease involves the islet cells. These cells are part of the pancreatic endocrine system and are spread all over the pancreas in clusters called islets of Langerhans. About 5 percent of the total pancreatic mass is made of endocrine cells. They cluster in groups that look like little islands when under a microscope; thus the name.

There are two types of islet cells. The alpha cells make glucagon, a hormone that raises the levels of glucose in the blood. The beta cells make insulin. Tumors of pancreatic islet cells, while rare, may manifest as sporadic tumors or as part of syndromes such as multiple endocrine neoplasia. They may be functional or nonfunctional. Functioning tumors produce excessive amounts of polypeptide hormones. They are usually small, and finding them can be a challenge to the radiologist. Nonfunctioning tumors are larger and are evident as a result of effects from their size or metastatic spread.

Tumors that arise from these islets also may produce a variety of hormones, though they don't all do that. Tumors can be benign or malignant, and symptoms are related to the particular type of hormone that the tumor is secreting. A family history of multiple endocrine neoplasia, type 1 (MEN1) is a risk for this type of cancer. Symptoms may include tremor, rapid heart beat, dizziness, behavioral changes, skin rash, weight loss, diarrhea, and abdominal pain.

Malignant tumors grow rapidly and spread to other organs. They can be viewed on ultrasound and need to be removed surgically. If the cancer has spread to the liver, part of that will need to be removed, too.

Chapter 9
The Liver

THE LIVER is the body's largest factory, providing for the synthesis of many compounds. It has a major role in the utilization of digested and absorbed nutrients. It is a source of energy production (power plant) for the body and an excretory organ to rid the body of waste products. Here are a few of its jobs:

- Regulates fat stores and controls production and release of cholesterol
- Changes the food you eat into energy, clotting factors, immune factors, hormones, and proteins
- Stores certain vitamins, minerals, sugars, and iron
- Breaks down drugs and medications and destroys poisonous substances
- Filters and detoxifies chemicals in what you eat, breathe, and absorb through the skin

It's no wonder that this large, multifunction organ can develop problems. Liver diseases are common and sometimes serious. Bile ducts can become blocked. Fat can accumulate. Genetic predispositions can skew metabolism. The liver can become infected, inflamed, and cirrhotic (irreparably scarred). In the following chapters in this section, you'll learn about these conditions and how to treat and prevent them.

The liver can regenerate. This is pointed out in the ancient Greek myth about Prometheus, one of four Titans born of Iapetus and Asia. When Prometheus insulted Zeus, Prometheus was chained to a rock to be tortured. Every day a great eagle would come to Prometheus and eat his liver, leaving only at nightfall, when the liver would begin to grow back, only to repeat the process again the next day.

In this chapter you will find information on:

- Hepatitis
- Primary biliary cirrhosis
- Primary sclerosing cholangitis
- Hemochromatosis
- Wilson's disease
- Alpha 1-antirypsin deficiency
- Steatosis and steatohepatitis: fatty liver
- Liver disease in pregnancy
- Benign liver tumors and masses
- Cirrhosis of the liver and liver failure
- Liver biopsy
- Liver tumors and liver cancer
- Liver transplantation

Hepatitis

Hepatitis is inflammation of the liver. Most of us know hepatitis as a disease one gets from contaminated water or shellfish, or as a sexually transmitted disease, or because of drug abuse with dirty needles. However, there are many types of hepatitis, and viral hepatitis (from A to E and even F and G) is only one of them. Viral hepatitis can also, less commonly, develop from Epstein-Barr virus (EBV, infectious mononucleosis) and the cytomegalovirus (CMV).

Some hepatitis is not caused by viruses but by other infectious agents, such as tuberculosis, malaria, amoebiasis, and bacteria from ascending cholangitis. There are autoimmune hepatitis and alcoholic hepatitis. Metabolic abnormalities also can lead to hepatitis, as can a fatty liver caused by obesity, diabetes, or alcoholism. Hepatitis also is related to toxic drugs such as cocaine; amphetamines; some cancer chemotherapy drugs; anti-HIV drugs; carbon tetrachloride; and even some herbal teas, such as Jamaican "bush tea" and comfrey, which are the most implicated.

Other forms of hepatitis may result from a side effect of commonly prescribed drugs and combinations of drugs, especially when people take several different types. The list of drugs that can be toxic to your liver is too long to include here, but it is important always to let any of your doctors know what medications you are taking. Some of the drugs that can be toxic include aspirin, penicillin, the anesthetic halothane, diazepam, and others.

Fulminant hepatitis is massive liver cell necrosis (death), and within days the entire liver can fail. This happens to less than 1 percent of people with viral hepatitis and also can result from medication (prescription and nonprescription). Acute hepatic failure can occur within weeks of onset. It is caused by infectious diseases, including viral; bacterial or parasitic infection; shock; acute fatty liver; toxic hepatitis; and other, rare conditions. It causes neurologic changes such as altered levels of consciousness, delirium, coma, and personality change. Other changes include bleeding, jaundice, and cardiopulmonary and renal failure. This can be fatal to the elderly and people who are in poor health. It usually results in consideration for liver transplantation.

Hepatitis can be acute or chronic if it lasts more than six months. With an acute condition the initial inflammation can be treated and run its course, but chronic hepatitis eventually damages the liver. Some patients progress to cirrhosis in five to ten years.

Viral Hepatitis

The hepatitis A and B viruses were identified after World War II. Then, in the 1970s, another form that didn't match either A or B was identified. It was called non-A or non-B, but once the viral genome was sequenced, it was named hepatitis C. Hepatitis D and E have been identified, but D needs the help of B to function.

Quite often, viral hepatitis is not diagnosed because the symptoms are vague and people think they are simply run down or have the flu. Some people have no symptoms at all, while others may have vomiting, nausea, diarrhea, muscle aches, and jaundice.

More than five million people in the United States are chronically infected with one form of viral hepatitis, according to the American Medical Association. Chronic viral hepatitis is the leading cause of chronic liver disease, liver cirrhosis, and liver cancer. Many more people contract the acute form of viral hepatitis, but fortunately they will recover and clear the virus. African Americans and Latinos have the highest rates of chronic viral hepatitis in the United States, especially in crowded urban environments with limited access to health care.

Hepatitis A   This is sometimes called infectious hepatitis and is generally spread by drinking water or eating food contaminated with human feces.

This type of hepatitis is not usually life-threatening. There are 10 million new cases reported globally every year. About 150,000 are in the United States, where there are 100 deaths. It can be prevented with a vaccine.

Hepatitis B   This is sometimes called serum hepatitis because it can be spread by blood transfusions, sexual contact, or from mother to child at birth. This can lead to cirrhosis. About 300 million people in the world are chronically infected, with 140,000 new cases in the United States every year. There are 1,000 deaths in the United States from Hepatitis B virus-related liver cancer. It can be prevented with a vaccine.

Hepatitis C   This is the most common form of viral hepatitis. It affects 170 million people worldwide, and 2.7 million in the United States. It is spread through contaminated blood and needles, but for many people the cause is still unknown. There are about 4 million people in the United States chronically infected with hepatitis C, with 35,000 new cases each year. About 9,000 people die from it each year in the United States. There is no vaccine to prevent it.

Hepatitis D   This is the form of viral hepatitis most often found in drug users who are also infected with the hepatitis B virus. This virus affects only those who simultaneously have hepatitis B and is a serious health problem. Most people with hepatitis D will progress to cirrhosis. Vaccination against hepatitis B will prevent hepatitis B and D.

Hepatitis E   This is similar to hepatitis A and is most often found in people who live in areas with poor sanitation. Virtually all cases of acute hepatitis E in the United States have been reported among travelers returning from developing countries with inadequate environmental sanitation where the disease is common. No vaccines are available to prevent the Hepatitis E virus.

Hepatitis F and hepatitis G   These are recently discovered viruses. The first report came from India in 1983, with subsequent reports from Europe and Japan. In 1987 it was named hepatitis F. In 1995 and 1996 two independent groups discovered and sequenced an agent similar to hepatitis C virus and named it hepatitis G. The G infection is transmitted by blood transfusion and is common in 1 to 2 percent of blood donors in the United States.

Hepatitis A

Hepatitis A (HAV) is a common cause of acute hepatitis but does not lead to chronic hepatitis. It tends to be self-limiting, meaning it can do only so much damage before it goes away. The infection in the liver is excreted into the bile and passed unharmed through the intestine, to be excreted through the feces up to three to four weeks after exposure. It has the highest transmission in areas of poor sanitation and hygiene.

HAV usually is transmitted through contaminated food such as raw shellfish or unclean drinking water. The virus is transmitted from person to person through oral or fecal contact with someone who has the disease, including food handlers and children in day-care centers. In developing countries, where the entire population is exposed to such contamination, people have developed antibodies in their immune systems that protect them. Before outsiders travel to such countries, they need to be vaccinated.

Symptoms and Diagnosis of Hepatitis A

Initial symptoms of HAV are flulike, with fatigue, fever, abdominal pain, vomiting, and jaundice. Dark urine usually precedes the jaundice. Symptoms usually peak in four to five weeks. The liver is slightly enlarged. Blood tests identify infection with virus.

Treating and Preventing Hepatitis A

There is no specific therapy, and most people recover completely from HAV within three months. Hepatitis A virus infection does not lead to chronic liver disease. An immune globulin (providing temporary immunity) prevents the disease 85 percent of the time when given within two weeks of exposure. Vaccines such as Havrix, Vaqta, Avaxim, Expaxal, and Twinrix prevent hepatitis A. These are pre-exposure prophylactics. Everyone at risk for contracting HAV should be vaccinated. This includes:

- Children living in communities with high HAV rates
- Anyone living with someone who has the disease
- International travelers to regions of endemic disease
- Homosexual men with multiple sex partners
- Injection drug users
- People exposed to nonhuman primates
- Staff members of chronic health-care and intensive-care facilities
- People with chronic liver disease
- Food handlers

Adults need two injections of vaccine in a six-to-twelve-month period for protection that lasts for ten years. Children from two to eighteen get two shots over a year. Supportive therapy may include bed rest, abstinence from alcohol, intravenous fluids, and vitamin K if blood clotting problems develop. If you have the disease, don't handle food. It is spread by eating food prepared by someone with the disease. Wash your hands frequently. Drink bottled water, and don't use ice cubes, fresh fruit, or vegetables in countries where hepatitis A is endemic.

For information about vaccination call your local or state health department or the Centers for Disease Control and Prevention (CDC). The CDC phone number is 1-800-232-2522. The CDC hepatitis Web site is www.cdc.gov/ncidod/diseases/hepatitis/hepatitis.htm. The National Immunization Program Web site is www.cdc.gov/nip.

Hepatitis B

Hepatitis B (HBV) accounts for 10 percent of chronic liver disease and cirrhosis in the United States. It is a major cause of liver cancer (especially worldwide) and is a completely preventable disease by vaccination of those at risk.

Most adults can get rid of the virus, but babies who are infected at birth progress to chronic infection at a higher rate. Hepatitis B is considered a sexually transmitted disease (STD) that can be contracted through intercourse and is a hundred times more infectious than HIV. Hepatitis D virus (HDV) is an incomplete virus that can coinfect those with hepatitis B infection and can severely exacerbate chronic hepatitis. (Hepatitis B vaccine will thus prevent two viral liver diseases, hepatitis B and hepatitis D.) About 80 percent of people who get HDV will progress to cirrhosis.

Transmission of hepatitis B is through blood and body fluids. High concentrations of the virus are found in blood, serum, and fluids from open wounds. Concentrations are moderate in semen, vaginal fluid, and saliva and low in urine, feces, sweat, tears, and breast milk.

Transmission of HBV is common from:

- Sex with an infected person without using a condom
- Sharing drug needles
- Getting a tattoo or body piercing with dirty tools used on others
- Getting pricked with a needle that has infected blood (e.g., involving health-care workers)
- Sharing a toothbrush or razor with an infected person

Symptoms and Diagnosis of Hepatitis B

Symptoms are similar to those of HAV, with flulike malaise and jaundice. A blood test will identify acute or chronic infection with the virus.

Treating and Preventing Hepatitis B

The goal of treatment is to wipe out the virus, decrease liver injury and fibrosis, and abolish the risk of developing cirrhosis. Treatment with interferon alpha injections takes six months but may help only 20 percent of patients. It works best with low virus levels but is not effective for people with cirrhosis. It also has toxic side effects.

Lamivudine, another drug to treat hepatitis B, is taken by mouth once a day for a year. Sometimes it is combined with interferon, but the combined effects are no better than either drug by itself. More than half the people who take lamivudine develop resistance to the drug in three years. However, it is a good drug for those with chronic liver disease. Side effects are fatigue, headache, fever, abdominal pain, myopathy, and neuropathy.

Adefovir dipivoxil is a new and effective drug. High doses cause renal toxicity, but it may be effective in people who develop resistance to lamivudine. Famciclovir and emtricitabine also show promise.

Vaccinations with hepatitis B vaccine are extremely effective in preventing HBV. All infants should be vaccinated with a series of three shots. So should anyone at risk, including people with HIV. Global and universal use of HBV vaccine is being investigated to see if we can eradicate this virus from the planet.

Hepatitis C

Hepatitis C (HCV) is the major cause of chronic hepatitis in developed countries. About 80 percent of people exposed to HCV will develop a chronic form of the infection, and it is the cause of about half the cases of liver cancer in the developed world. Before better testing procedures in hospitals, it was mostly associated with blood transfusions. Now it is primarily contracted by alcoholics, people with STDs, intravenous drug abusers, and people who use cocaine through the nose. About 60 percent of this disease is among intravenous drug users. Sex accounts for about 15 percent. Babies born to infected mothers, hemophiliacs, and those on hemodialysis also are at risk. About 25 percent of HIV-infected people in the United States also have HCV, and the hepatitis infection progresses more rapidly to liver damage in these cases.

Despite screening of blood products and other interventions resulting in a significant reduction of acute hepatitis C in the United States and elsewhere, there remains a large reservoir of chronically infected people, many of whom are unaware of their infection. Some of these cases are detected on routine physical examinations.

Like hepatitis B, with which it can coexist, hepatitis C can lead to cancer, but there is up to a thirty-year period of latency. About a third of chronic patients will develop serious liver disease and cirrhosis over twenty years, and some will require a transplant. In fact, HCV is the primary indication for liver transplant in the United States (Transplantation is discussed later in this chapter.)

Chronic hepatitis C varies greatly in its course and outcome. At one end of the spectrum are people who have no signs or symptoms of liver disease and completely normal levels of liver enzymes in their blood. Liver biopsy usually shows some degree of chronic hepatitis, but the degree of injury usually is mild and the overall prognosis is good. At the other end are those with severe hepatitis C who have symptoms, the virus in their blood, elevated liver enzymes, and who ultimately develop cirrhosis and end-stage liver disease. In the middle are those with few or no symptoms and an uncertain prognosis.

A few people develop complications that do not involve the liver, such as skin rashes, kidney disease, neuropathy, and other conditions. Diseases well documented to be associated to hepatitis C include fibromyalgia, non-Hodgkin's lymphoma, and arthritis.

Symptoms and Diagnosis of Hepatitis C

Mild symptoms of HCV occur within seven to eight weeks of exposure and include fatigue, tenderness in the upper right abdomen, nausea, poor appetite, and muscle and joint pain. Symptoms are more prominent as the disease becomes severe and also may include weight loss, dark urine, fluid retention, and abdominal swelling.

Diagnosis is based on symptoms and blood tests. Detecting the hepatitis C virus in the blood is not always easy and often will not show up until two to eight weeks after the onset of symptoms. Testing for HCV RNA is helpful. This test looks directly for viral particles in the blood. The test is repeated a month later. Diagnosis must include ruling out other forms of hepatitis. Hepatitis C genotyping also can be done with blood tests to help determine the likelihood of treatment response. Clinical examination may find an enlarged liver and spleen, jaundice, muscle wasting, ankle swelling, and ascites (fluid in the peritoneal cavity). Only a liver biopsy can accurately stage the disease and determine the presence of fibrosis, inflammation, and iron deposits, check for coexistence with other liver disease, and guide decisions for therapy.

Treating Hepatitis C

Dual therapy with interferon and ribavarin is most effective in people who are young and who do not have cirrhosis. If treatment begins within months of infection, it can lead to complete cure. However, many people do not tolerate a forty-eight week course of the full dose. Interferon drugs have a short life, and combined with the speed of the HCV virus in replicating itself, this therapy is not always effective. There are several types of interferon, including long-acting forms (peg interferon), which requires only weekly injections.

Interferon can cause flulike symptoms early in treatment, but these diminish as treatment continues. Later side effects may include fatigue; hair loss; low blood count; moodiness; and depression, which needs to be monitored closely. As many as 40 percent of people treated with this drug may suffer severe side effects. Rare side effects include diabetes mellitus, retinopathy, hearing impairment, or seizures. Treatment may need to be stopped in as many as 15 percent. Pregnant women should not use it at all because of potential birth defects.

Likewise, ribavarin may cause anemia, a rash, and in pregnant women, birth defects.

Nonviral Hepatitis

Hepatitis also can develop from alcohol and drugs, including common medications. Autoimmune disease also can cause hepatitis.

Drug-Induced Hepatitis

Drug induced hepatitis also is known as toxic hepatitis. Liver inflammation is caused by drugs, alcohol, and medications. This type has similar symptoms as viral hepatitis including nausea, jaundice, and fatigue.

Analgesics and antipyretics that contain acetaminophen (such as Tylenol) are a common cause of liver inflammation. This is a good reason never to take a higher-than-recommended dose of over-the-counter analgesics and antipyretics that contain acetaminophen. If you drink regularly or heavily, avoid these drugs altogether.

Be careful of all drugs that may contain acetaminophen. In addition to Tylenol, these drugs contain it:

- Percocet
- Vicodin
- Four-way Cold
- Bayer Select Flu Relief

- Benedryl Cold
- Comtrex Hot Flu Relief
- Dristan Cold and Flu
- Vicks NyQuil Liquicaps
- Robitussin Honey Flu
- Vicks DayQuil Liquicaps
- Aspirin-Free Excedrin Caplets
- Anacin-3
- Dorcol Children's Fever and Pain Reducer
- Feverall Children's
- Infants' Anacin-3
- St. Joseph's Aspirin-Free Fever Reducer for Children

Other problem drugs include the general anesthetic halothane; methyldopa; isoniazid (used to treat TB); methotrexate; amiodarone; and HMG CoA reductase inhibitors, which also are called statins. Statins are cholesterol-lowering drugs. One of them, Baycol, was pulled from the market because of numerous deaths associated with its use. If you are taking prescribed cholesterol-lowering medications, your doctor should be monitoring your liver to watch for any indication of toxicity. Statins available in the United States include:

- Lipitor
- Zocor
- Pravachol
- Lescol
- Mevacor
- Crestor

Some medications interfere with the flow of bile. These include erythromycin, oral contraceptives, chlorpromazine, and anabolic steroids. Anyone with a history of liver problems should avoid these drugs:

- Isoniazid
- Oral contraceptives
- Androgens
- Chlorpromazine, oral
- Chlorpromazine, injectable

- Allopurinol, oral
- Acetaminophen
- Hydralazine, oral
- Halothane
- Valproic acid
- Phenytoin
- Carbamazepine, oral
- Methotrexate
- 6-mercaptopurine

Herbal teas used for a variety of complaints may also have a negative effect on the liver. In addition to Jamaican bush tea these include tea from germander blossoms, chaparral used in the American southwest, and Jin Bu Huan, a Chinese herbal sedative and pain reliever. Chaparral, a desert shrub, has a long history as a traditional medicine among Native Americans. At least six cases of acute non-viral hepatitis have been associated with this tea and more cases are under investigation. Comfrey contains pyrrolizidine alkaloids and its toxicity to humans is well documented. In France, at least one death and a dozen cases of acute nonviral hepatitis have been connected to commercially available germander products. Germander contains several chemicals including polyphenols, tannins, diterpenoids, and flavonoids.

Symptoms and Diagnosis of Drug-Induced Hepatitis

Symptoms of drug-induced hepatitis are similar to those caused by viral hepatitis, including jaundice and nausea, but some people may have no symptoms. These usually are people who are noted to have a mild elevation in their liver enzymes (found on blood testing), which results in a search for the cause.

Treating and Preventing Drug-Induced Hepatitis

Once the drug is stopped, the hepatitis usually subsides within days or weeks. When symptoms are severe, rest and avoid physical exertion, alcohol, and any drugs mentioned. If nausea and vomiting are significant, you may need to consider intravenous fluids to avoid dehydration.

Alcoholic Hepatitis

Alcoholic hepatitis is drug-induced. Alcohol is ethanol, a chemical that can alter the activity of enzymes that transport proteins.

In Western societies, alcohol abuse is the most common cause of serious liver disease. It affects about 1 percent of the population. Since the 1960s, death rates due to alcoholic hepatitis have been greater for the nonwhite population than for the white population.

There is evidence of a genetic predilection to alcoholism, but the role of genetic factors in susceptibility to alcoholic liver injury is much less clear. Most alcoholics do not develop severe liver injury. However, gender clearly affects susceptibility. For a given level of ethanol intake, women are more susceptible than men to alcoholic liver disease.

Alcohol rehabilitation is a major part of treatment. Once consumption of alcohol ceases, treatment focuses on replacing nutritional and vitamin deficiencies. Most people with alcohol hepatitis show protein calorie malnutrition (PCM), and many have high iron deposits in the liver that need to be treated.

Use of medications in alcoholic hepatitis remains controversial. Despite decades of research and multiple clinical trials, only glucocorticoid (steroid) treatment can be considered of probable benefit, and only for people with severe alcoholic hepatitis. Glucocorticoid (steroids) may increase complications and mortality associated with GI bleeding, pancreatitis, and other conditions.

Autoimmune Hepatitis

Autoimmune diseases such as lupus and rheumatoid arthritis are caused by the body's own immune system attacking itself. In autoimmune hepatitis, it attacks the liver cells, causing inflammation. A genetic factor is believed to predispose some people to autoimmune diseases. Women between ages fifteen and forty account for about 70 percent of this type of hepatitis. However, in the older age groups, men are more commonly affected than women. Prevalence is greatest among northern European Caucasians. The disease usually is detected in the third to fifth decade of life, but young children and older adults also may be affected.

Scientists suspect that certain bacteria, viruses, toxins, and drugs trigger an autoimmune response in people who are genetically susceptible to an autoimmune disorder. Autoimmune hepatitis usually is quite serious; unless it is treated it becomes chronic, eventually leading to cirrhosis and liver failure.

There are two types of autoimmune hepatitis. Type I is the most common form in North America, and about half the people who have this type have other autoimmune disorders, such as thyroidosis, Graves' disease, Sjögren's syndrome, autoimmune anemia, and ulcerative colitis.

Type I occurs at any age. Type II is less common, typically affecting girls from two to fourteen, although adults can have it, too.

Autoimmune hepatitis is now recognized as a multisystem disorder that can coexist with other liver diseases, such as chronic viral hepatitis, and also may be triggered by certain viral infections such as hepatitis A, or chemicals such as minocycline, a form of tetracycline, that sometimes is used in the treatment of adolescent acne.

Symptoms and Diagnosis of Autoimmune Hepatitis

Symptoms of autoimmune hepatitis can be mild or severe, with fatigue the most common. Other symptoms include enlarged liver, jaundice, itching, skin rashes, joint pain, and abdominal discomfort. In the advanced stages of this hepatitis, fluid builds up in the abdomen (ascites). Mental confusion can occur, and women may stop having menstrual periods.

Because severe viral hepatitis and drug-induced hepatitis have the same symptoms as autoimmune hepatitis, a careful diagnosis must rule out these forms of the disease. Prescription and over-the-counter medications must be taken into account for any possible role in the disease. Blood tests for liver enzymes can help reveal a pattern typical of autoimmune hepatitis and distinguish it from other types of hepatitis. Tests for autoantibodies also are needed. The immune system makes antibodies to fight off bacteria and viruses. In some autoimmune hepatitis, the immune system makes a variety of antibodies. The pattern level of these antibodies helps define the type of autoimmune hepatitis, either I or II.

A liver biopsy (discussed later in this chapter) can help pinpoint this type of hepatitis and detect how advanced it is.

Treating Autoimmune Hepatitis

When autoimmune hepatitis is diagnosed early, it usually can be controlled. Recent studies show that sustained response to treatment not only stops the disease from getting worse but may actually reverse some of the damage. Medication can slow down an overactive immune system. Prednisone, a corticosteroid, may begin at high daily levels and then decrease to the lowest possible dose to control the disease. Imuran (azathioprine) also is used, sometimes along with prednisone. Like prednisone, it suppresses the immune system, but in a different way. The combination allows a smaller dose of prednisone, thereby reducing the side effects of that drug. Treatment with prednisone, with or without azathioprine, may be needed for years; even for life. Everyone responds differently to medications. In about one of every three people, treatment can eventually be stopped within two years. Some will see the disease return within three years, so treatment may be necessary on and off, for years.

Careful monitoring must continue after treatment, so any new symptoms can be reported. The disease can return and be even more severe, especially in the few months after stopping treatment.

People with acute autoimmune hepatitis and symptoms of nausea and vomiting may require intravenous fluids and even total parenteral nutrition. However, most people can tolerate a regular diet. If ascites (abdominal fluid) has developed, then a low-salt diet may be advisable.

Side effects   Because high doses of prednisone are needed to control the disease, managing side effects is very important. Both prednisone and azathioprine have side effects. Azathioprine can lower the white blood cell count and sometimes causes nausea and poor appetite. It can cause allergic reaction, liver damage, or pancreatitis, but these are very rare. Most side effects appear only after a long period of time. They include weight gain, anxiety and confusion, osteoporosis, diabetes, high blood pressure, cataracts, and thinning of the hair and skin. If the side effects are too severe or therapy doesn't work, immunosuppressive agents such as cyclosporine or tacrolimus can be used. If the disease has already caused liver failure, then liver transplantation (see later in this chapter) may be necessary.

Cholestatic and Metabolic Liver Diseases

Cholestatic liver disease develops when there are high levels of bile acids in the liver, possibly because of gallstones, pregnancy, oral contraceptives, or drugs such as tetracyclines. It may be induced by inflammatory disease such as primary biliary cirrhosis or sclerosing cholangitis, which attacks the bile ducts. Biliary congestions or biliary sludge also can cause it. And in some people it is inherited. Cholestatic liver disease may progress to cirrhosis.

Symptoms include pruritus (intense itching of the skin with no eruption), and jaundice from too much bilirubin, a waste product resulting from the breakdown of worn out red blood cells, and that is normally excreted from the body. It stains fatty tissue yellow, and thus jaundice occurs. To diagnose correctly, other diseases need to be ruled out.

Primary Biliary Cirrhosis

Primary biliary cirrhosis (PBC), a chronic progressive destruction of the bile ducts and eventual destruction of the liver, usually affects middle-aged women (90 percent). PBC is more prevalent in the United Kingdom and Scandinavia. Bile metabolizes fat, and when the ducts are damaged, bile builds up in the liver and damages tissue. Over time the disease can cause cirrhosis and liver failure. The cause and why it affects women is unknown. Some research suggests that it might be caused by a problem within the immune system.

Symptoms and Diagnosis of Primary Biliary Cirrhosis

The most common symptoms of PBC are fatigue and pruritus. Other symptoms include cholesterol deposits on the skin, fluid retention, and dry eyes or mouth. By the time jaundice occurs, the disease has progressed to end stages. Some people with primary biliary cirrhosis also have osteoporosis, arthritis, or thyroid problems. It is diagnosed through blood tests, X-rays, CT, sonograms, and in some cases liver biopsy. Elevated bilirubin levels often show up without jaundice.

Treating Primary Biliary Cirrhosis

Ursodiol is used to treat primary biliary cirrhosis, although it does not cure the disease. Another drug, Questran, helps bile salt absorption and also lowers cholesterol. Phenobarbital stimulates bile flow. Some therapies appear to slow progression, but most patients eventually have liver failure and need a transplant. Ultraviolet light, vitamin and calcium supplements, and hormone therapy can relieve symptoms. Baths with colloidal oatmeal often reduce pruritus.

Primary Sclerosing Cholangitis

Unlike primary biliary cirrhosis, primary sclerosing cholangitis (PSC) affects mostly men. It is a chronic cholestatic liver disease that is probably an autoimmune condition. It is associated with inflammatory bowel disease (IBD) 75 percent of the time. And of these cases, 90 percent have ulcerative colitis. The rest have Crohn's disease and nearly always Crohn's colitis. The association with IBD makes the autoimmune connection more likely.

PSC mainly affects young adults, with the average age of forty, more than half of them men, but it can arise in childhood. It progresses so slowly that people have it for years without knowing. As the bile ducts inside and outside the liver become inflamed and scarred, they become blocked and can no longer carry bile out of the liver. If ducts are blocked, bile builds up in the liver and damages the cells. Eventually this can cause liver failure.

PSC can occur even in people who have had their colon removed. Inflammatory cells from the intestines migrate to and remain in the liver.

Infectious triggers in the gut or liver may stimulate the disease process. Toxins such as chemotherapy and bone marrow transplantation also may be implicated.

Symptoms and Diagnosis of Primary Sclerosing Cholangitis

The main symptoms of primary sclerosing cholangitis are itching, fatigue, and jaundice. An infection of the bile ducts can cause chills and fever. Other liver function abnormalities may be present.

Diagnosis is done through cholangiography, which involves injecting dye into the bile ducts and then taking an X-ray. This can be performed as an endoscopic procedure, through radiology or surgery, or with MRI scans (see chapter 3).

Treating Primary Sclerosing Cholangitis

Treatment includes medication to relieve itching, antibiotics for infection, and vitamin supplements. People with PSC are usually deficient in vitamins A, D, E, and K. In some cases, surgery or interventional radiology procedures are necessary to open major blockages in the common bile duct. PSC can be controlled for some time, but if the disease advances, the liver fails and transplantation is necessary. You'll find more about transplantation later in this chapter.

Metabolic Liver Diseases

The liver is the metabolism processing plant in your body. If the mechanism of this action should break down or is genetically faulty, then a number of conditions can result. Your body may have problems metabolizing iron or copper and certain other critical substances, as well as fat. Selected enzyme deficiencies are another cause of metabolic liver diseases.

Hemochromatosis

Hemochromatosis is the most common form of iron overload disease. When iron is not metabolized by the liver, it gets deposited abnormally in many sites and causes problems in other organs. This can cause cirrhosis, diabetes, skin pigmentation, endocrine failure, adrenal insufficiency (hypogonadism), hypothyroidism, cardiac abnormalities, and joint diseases.

Iron is an essential nutrient found in many foods, including red meat and iron-fortified bread and cereal. In the body, iron becomes part of hemoglobin, a molecule in the blood that transports oxygen from the lungs to all body tissues. Normally, about 10 percent of the iron contained in the food we eat is absorbed to meet the body's needs. However, someone with hemochromatosis absorbs more iron than the body needs. And since the body has no natural way to rid itself of excess iron, it is stored in body tissues, especially the liver, heart, and pancreas. Without treatment, hemochromatosis can cause these organs to fail.

Hemochromatosis is mostly hereditary, but if the liver has been damaged by other diseases, it can develop simply because the liver cannot do its job in processing iron. In the United States, the primary overload cause in some is genetically determined. Men develop this condition with cirrhosis and diabetes more often than women. Alcoholism increases iron deposits in the liver, for example. In women the disease is more commonly manifest with skin pigmentation and fatigue. Women have less blood volume than men to begin with, have less iron in their diet, and they loose blood and iron through menstruation. Women have significantly lower mean concentrations of iron than men. Surveys in Australia and New Zealand and other industrialized countries report that many adolescent girls have dietary intakes of iron and zinc that fail to meet their high physiologic requirements for growing body tissue, expanding red cell mass, and the onset of menarche. Some dietary inadequacies can be attributed to poor food selection patterns and low energy intake.

Hereditary Hemochromatosis

Iron stores in the body are highly regulated and sensed by intestinal crypt cells. A defect in a gene called HFE, which helps regulate the amount of iron absorbed from food, is associated with hereditary hemochromatosis. There are two known mutations in HFE, named C282Y and H63D. C282Y is the more important. When that mutation is inherited from both parents, too much iron is absorbed from the diet. H63D usually causes little increase in iron absorption. However, a person with H63D from one parent and C282Y from the other may develop hemochromatosis, but this is very rare.

While the genetic defect is present at birth, symptoms rarely appear before adulthood. If you inherit the defective gene from both parents, you may develop hemochromatosis, but if you inherit it from only one parent, you are a carrier for the disease but won't get it yourself. Carriers, however, may have a slight increase in iron absorption.

Hereditary hemochromatosis is one of the most common genetic disorders in the United States, most often affecting Caucasians of northern European descent. About five in every thousand Caucasians here carry two copies of the hemochromatosis gene and are susceptible to developing the disease. One person in eight to twelve is a carrier of the abnormal gene. Hemochromatosis is less common in African Americans, Asian Americans, Hispanic Americans, and Native Americans. (However, in sub-Saharan Africa, iron absorbed from home-brewed beer made in iron vats has caused hemochromatosis.)

Although both men and women can inherit the gene defect, men are about five times more likely to be diagnosed with the effects of hereditary hemochromatosis than women. Men also tend to develop problems from the excess iron at a younger age.

Nonhereditary Hemochromatosis

Juvenile hemochromatosis and neonatal hemochromatosis are two forms of the disease that are not caused by an HFE defect and whose cause is unknown. The juvenile form leads to severe iron overload and liver and heart disease in adolescents and young adults between fifteen and thirty. The neonatal form causes the same problems in newborns.

Symptoms and Diagnosis of Hemochromatosis

By the time symptoms drive someone to see a doctor, hemochromatosis is fairly well established. Symptoms tend to occur in men between ages thirty and fifty and in women over fifty. However, many people have no symptoms, and they are diagnosed while getting routine blood tests.

Hemochromatosis is often undiagnosed and untreated because it is considered rare and doctors may not think to test for it. The initial symptoms can be diverse and vague and mimic the symptoms of many other diseases. Also, doctors may focus on conditions caused by hemochromatosis—arthritis, liver disease, heart disease, or diabetes—rather than the underlying iron overload. However, if the iron overload caused by hemochromatosis is diagnosed and treated before organ damage has occurred, a person can live a normal, healthy life.

A thorough medical history, physical examination, and routine blood tests help rule out other conditions that could be causing the symptoms of hemochromatosis. This information often provides helpful clues, such as a family history of arthritis or unexplained liver disease.

Blood tests can determine whether the amount of iron stored in the body is too high. The transferring saturation test determines how much iron is bound to the protein that carries iron in the blood. The serum ferritin test shows the level of iron in the liver. If either of these tests shows higher-than-normal levels of iron in the body, doctors can order a special blood test to detect the HFE gene mutation, which will help confirm the diagnosis. If the mutation is not present, then doctors will look for other causes of the iron buildup. A liver biopsy (discussed later in this chapter) may be needed to show how much iron has accumulated in the liver and whether the liver is damaged.

Complications of Hemochromatosis

If hemochromatosis is not detected and treated early, iron accumulation in body tissues may eventually lead to serious problems, such as:

- Arthritis and joint pain
- Liver disease, including enlarged liver, cirrhosis, cancer, and liver failure
- Damage to the pancreas
- Heart abnormalities such as irregular heart rhythms or congestive heart failure
- Impotence
- Early menopause
- Abnormal pigmentation of the skin, making it look gray or bronze
- Thyroid deficiency
- Damage to adrenal glands

Treating Hemochromatosis

Hemochromatosis usually is treated by a gastroenterologist, a hepatologist (a specialist in liver disorders), or a hematologist (a specialist in blood disorders). Because of other problems associated with the condition, several other specialists may be part of the treatment team. People who have complications of hemochromatosis may want to consider getting treatment from one of the specialized hemochromatosis centers located throughout the country.

Treatment is simple, inexpensive, and safe, and the goal is first to rid the body of excess iron. This is done with phlebotomy, a process for removing blood. Depending on how severe the iron overload is, a pint of blood will be taken once or twice a week for several months to a year, and occasionally longer. Blood ferritin tests monitor iron levels periodically. Depending on the amount of iron overload at diagnosis, reaching normal levels can take many phlebotomies. Once iron levels return to normal, maintenance therapy involves giving a pint of blood every two to four months for life. Some may need it more often. An annual blood ferritin test will help determine how often blood should be removed.

The earlier hemochromatosis is diagnosed and treated, the better. If treatment begins before any organs are damaged, associated conditions can be prevented. The outlook for people who already have these conditions at diagnosis depends on the degree of organ damage. For example, treating hemochromatosis can stop the progression of liver disease in its early stages, which means normal life expectancy. However, if cirrhosis has developed, the risk of developing liver cancer increases, even if iron stores are reduced to normal levels.

If you have hemochromatosis, do not take iron supplements or eat food high in iron such as red meat and organ meets. Avoid drinking alcohol because that causes further damage to the liver. Although treatment cannot cure the conditions associated with hemochromatosis, it will help most of them. The main exception is arthritis, which may not improve even when excess iron is removed from the blood.

Screening for and Prevention of Hemochromatosis

Everyone should be screened for iron levels at least once in a lifetime. Serum iron and transferrin saturation levels should be measured. If the tests are abnormal, then a needle liver biopsy (discussed later in this chapter) should be done. Screening for hemochromatosis is not a routine part of medical care or checkups, but researchers and public health officials do have some suggestions.

- Brothers and sisters of people who have hemochromatosis should have their blood tested to see if they have the disease or are carriers.

- Parents, children, and other close relatives of people who have the disease should consider testing.

- Doctors should consider testing people who have joint disease, severe and continuing fatigue, heart disease, elevated liver enzymes, impotence, or diabetes, because these conditions may result from hemochromatosis.

Since the genetic defect is common and early detection and treatment are so effective, some researchers and advocacy groups want widespread screening of hemochromatosis. However, a simple, inexpensive, and accurate test does not yet exist, and the available options have limitations. For example, the genetic test provides a definitive diagnosis, but it is expensive. The blood test for transferring saturation is widely available and relatively inexpensive, but it may have to be done twice with careful handling to confirm a diagnosis and to show that it is a consequence of iron overload.

Scientists hope that further study of the HFE gene will reveal how the body normally metabolizes iron. They also want to learn how iron injures cells and whether it contributes to organ damage in other diseases, such as alcoholic liver disease, hepatitis C, porphyria cutanea tarda, heart disease, reproductive disorders, cancer, autoimmune hepatitis, diabetes, and joint disease.

These organizations provide information:

American Hemochromatosis Society, Inc., at www.americanhs.org or phone 1-888-655-IRON (4766)

American Liver Foundation at www.liverfoundation.org or phone 1-800-465-4837

Hemochromatosis Foundation, Inc., at www.hemochromatosis.org or phone 518-489-0972

National Organization of Rare Disorders, Inc. (NORD), at www.rarediseases.org or phone 1-800-999-6673

Wilson's Disease

Just as hemochromatosis causes the body to retain iron, Wilson's disease (WD) is a hereditary condition that causes the body to retain copper. The intestines absorb copper from food and it builds up in the liver, which does not release the copper into the bile, as it should. Eventually the damage causes the liver to release the copper directly into the bloodstream and it circulates throughout the body. When copper builds up in the body it can damage kidneys, brain, and eyes. If not treated, Wilson's disease can cause severe brain damage, liver failure, and death.

Copper is a trace mineral found in oysters, lobsters, and other shellfish. Very small amounts are found in potatoes, avocados, and a few other foods. Copper also is included in many multivitamins. It also may leach into drinking water in buildings with copper pipes. We need only a minute amount in our diet, but with Wilson's disease, even such minute amounts add up when they are not eliminated.

An American neurologist, Samuel Alexander Kinnier Wilson, first described WD in 1912, characterizing the disease as a degenerative central nervous disorder associated with a cirrhotic liver.

Approximately one in every thirty thousand people in the United States has WD, and one in every ninety is a carrier. The disease is found in every ethnic and geographic population, and men and women are affected equally. Higher frequencies are encountered in inbred populations of Sardinia and several Japanese islands. People younger than twenty usually discover the disease because of liver problems, but in adults, the initial findings usually are neurologic or psychiatric in nature.

WD is similar to a disease called copper toxicosis (CT), which is found in Bedlington terriers. This is one reason why CT was one of the first genetic diseases to be part of a DNA study. There had already been so much research done with the human disease that researchers were hoping the DNA information would easily transfer.

Symptoms and Diagnosis of Wilson's Disease

Symptoms of Wilson's disease usually appear between ages six and twenty but can begin as late as forty. The most characteristic sign is the Kayser-Fleischer ring—a greenish brown ring of copper deposited around the cornea of the eye. Other symptoms depend on whether the damage occurs in the liver, blood, central nervous system, urinary system, or musculoskeletal system. Some symptoms are obvious, such as jaundice or vomiting blood. Speech and language problems, tremors in the arms and hands, and rigid muscles also are signs. Many signs or symptoms of Wilson's disease can be detected only by a doctor, such as swelling of the liver and spleen; fluid buildup in the lining of the abdomen; anemia; low platelet and white blood cell count in the blood; high levels of amino acids, protein, uric acid, and carbohydrates in urine; and softening of the bones.

Wilson's disease is diagnosed through tests that measure the amount of copper in the blood, urine, and liver. An eye exam would detect the Kayser-Fleischer ring.

Treating Wilson's Disease

Wilson's disease is treated with lifelong use of drugs to help remove copper from the body: D-penicillamine or trientine hydrochloride. Zinc acetate, another drug used in treatment, stops the intestines from absorbing copper and helps the body excrete the copper. Vitamin B_6 and a low-copper diet are recommended. If the disorder is detected early and treated correctly, you can enjoy a completely normal life.

For more information, contact the Wilson's Disease Association at www.wilsonsdisease.org or phone 1-800-399-0266.

Alpha 1-Antitrypsin Deficiency

Alpha 1-antitrypsin (also called AAT or alpha 1 proteinase inhibitor) is a protein produced in the liver that is designed to protect the lungs from bacteria and aging and provide for healing. A deficiency of this protein is a rare hereditary defect that fewer than a hundred thousand Americans have. Some people who do not have the genetic predisposition can develop this deficiency when they have a cirrhotic liver, which can no longer produce the protein.

AAT helps prevent certain white blood cell enzymes (proteinases) from going beyond their regular infection-fighting functions to attack healthy body tissue. When the body doesn't make enough AAT, the lungs often don't work as efficiently, and the liver may be adversely affected. Over the years, this deficiency can result in emphysema and also can put a mild strain on the liver. Problems in the liver usually begin just after birth or not until middle age.

This genetic defect is similar to the way hemochromatosis is inherited. If one parent has it, the child will be a carrier. If both parents have it, the child will most likely get it. It is a good idea to get tested for this deficiency before having children. If the defect is already present, it is really important to refrain from smoking. This is the single most important way to protect the health of your lungs.

The major manifestation of AAT deficiency in the first two decades of life is liver disease; pulmonary manifestations appear later. People with AAT deficiency frequently develop dyspnea (shortness of breath) twenty to thirty years earlier than smokers who have emphysema but don't have the AAT deficiency. A minority of patients develops hepatic cirrhosis.

Treating Alpha 1-Antitrypsin Deficiency

If recurrent episodes of cough are prominent, patients may be treated with multiple courses of antibiotics and evaluated for sinusitis, postnasal drip, or gastroesophageal reflux. By the time dyspnea becomes dominant and a diagnosis is established, most patients will have seen several physicians over several years.

Quitting smoking is mandatory to increase survival. The focus of treatment is to improve lung function with medications and prevent respiratory infections. Supplemental oxygen may be needed at intervals as well as weekly intravenous infusions of pooled human plasma alpha-1 antiprotease (called IV augmentation therapy, which has been widely available since 1989). The cost of therapy for people with alpha 1 antitrypsin deficiency is very high, whether or not they receive augmental therapy.

Steatosis and Steohepatitis: Fatty Liver

Fatty liver is called steatosis and is common in alcoholics. However, obese people develop this condition even if they don't drink. If the fatty liver is inflamed, it is called steatohepatitis. Steatohepatitis that is not caused by alcohol is sometimes referred to as nonalcoholic steatohepatitis or NASH.

Fat in the liver may not cause damage by itself, but is a sign of a problem because a buildup of fat in the liver cells is not normal. Just what determines who will develop fatty liver is not known. Some mildly obese and occasionally nonobese patients will develop fatty liver, while some who are obese will not. However, studies show that many significantly overweight people have developed or will develop steatohepatitis. It also can occur with rapid weight loss. Steatohepatitis has been connected to estrogen hormones in some women. Researchers believe it also may develop in people with uncontrolled diabetes. High blood triglycerides also may pose a risk.

Certain illnesses have been implicated in promoting a fatty liver, including tuberculosis, malnutrition, intestinal bypass surgery for obesity, and excess vitamin A in the body. The use of certain drugs such as Depakote and corticosteroids such as prednisone, also may promote fatty liver. Sometimes it is a complication of pregnancy. (See page 193).

Symptoms and Diagnosis of Steatosis and Steohepatitis

Fatty liver is frequently uncovered during a routine physical exam because there are no usual symptoms. There may be a rise in certain liver enzymes found in the blood, and sometimes the liver is slightly enlarged. An ultrasound exam of the abdomen may show fat in the liver. However, before an accurate diagnosis can be made, all other causes of hepatitis have to be excluded. A careful drug and alcohol history needs to be taken and blood tested for the hepatitis virus. Metabolic disease also must be ruled out. A liver biopsy would be needed to be certain.

Treating Steatosis and Steohepatitis

Weight loss is the most critical factor in ridding the liver of fat. This is especially critical if liver damage is occurring and early signs of scarring are present. Triglyceride levels and diabetes also are worse with obesity, so weight loss improves all conditions. It may be difficult to do, but the alternative is liver failure and the need for a transplant.

Weight reduction works, but most patients don't stick to the program. Three obese patients studied were treated for six months to a year with a weight reduction program, including the drug orlistat. Those who lost weight had significant improvement. Clofibrate, a drug known to lower lipids, has been used in clinical studies.

Some drugs such as ursodeoxycholic acid and Actigall, which are under study, appear to reduce the liver damage from steatohepatitis, but there is no certainty yet. Alphatocopherol is another drug used successfully.

Cirrhosis of the Liver and Liver Failure

Any of the liver conditions already covered in this book could lead to cirrhosis if they become chronic and are not properly treated. A cirrhotic liver is one that is so damaged that scar tissue predominates. Blood cannot flow through the scar tissue and therefore the liver cannot do its work. Cirrhosis is the eighth leading cause of death by disease in the United States, killing twenty-five thousand people each year. Most people associate cirrhosis with alcoholism, but alcohol is only one of the causes. In this country, chronic hepatitis C and alcoholism are the most common causes of cirrhosis. Other causes include:

- Hepatitis: Chronic hepatitis B and D are the most common cause of cirrhosis worldwide, but in the United States and other Western countries, it is less common.

- Autoimmune hepatitis

- Inherited diseases such as hemochromatosis, Wilson's disease, alpha-1 antitrypsin deficiency, and other rare conditions that interfere with liver function.

- Nonalcoholic steatohepatitis (NASH), also known as fatty liver, is associated with obesity, diabetes, protein malnutrition, coronary artery disease, and corticosteroid treatment. Fat builds up in the liver and may eventually cause scar tissue.

- Blocked bile ducts prevent bile from leaving the liver and therefore it backs up and damages the liver tissue. In adults, primary biliary cirrhosis is the most common cause of this condition.

- Severe reactions to prescription drugs. Cirrhosis prevents the liver from filtering medications from the blood. This means that the medications are in the bloodstream longer than usual and build up in the body. Someone then becomes more sensitive to the medication and the side effects, too.

- Parasitic infection of schistosomiasis. Although rare in this country, it is a serious problem in developing countries. It is contacted by ingesting infected freshwater snails; the parasite can survive and replicate in human hosts for years and even decades.

- Prolonged exposure to environmental toxins is a known cause, but there is speculation about just what toxins are at fault. It is known that the liver filters them. Agent Orange is one such controversial toxin.

- Repeated bouts of heart failure with liver congestion can lead to cirrhosis. Cardiac cirrhosis includes a spectrum of hepatic derangements that occur in the setting of right-sided heart failure. Clinically, the signs and symptoms of congestive heart failure dominate the disorder. Unlike cirrhosis caused by chronic alcohol use related to viral hepatitis, the effect of cardiac cirrhosis on overall prognosis is unknown.

Symptoms and Diagnosis of Cirrhosis of the Liver

In the early stages of cirrhosis, many people have no symptoms, but as scar tissue replaces healthy tissue, liver function begins to fail and symptoms develop. They include exhaustion, fatigue, loss of appetite, weakness, and weight loss. Complications develop as cirrhosis progresses; sometimes these symptoms may be the first hint of the disease. Other symptoms include:

- *Bruising and bleeding.* Certain proteins are needed to help the blood clot normally, and when the liver no longer produces them or slows down production, bruising and bleeding occur easily.

- *Jaundice.* When the skin and eyes turn yellow, it means the liver is not absorbing enough bilirubin because it is not functioning properly.

- *Gallstones.* These may develop in the bile ducts if a damaged liver prevents bile from reaching the gallbladder.

A doctor can palpate the liver to see if it is hard or enlarged, a sign of cirrhosis, but many more tests are needed for an accurate diagnosis. A medical history, description of symptoms, and a complete physical are the beginning. Blood tests will determine if liver disease is present. A CT scan, ultrasound, or laparoscope will allow a look at the liver for signs of scarring and disease. A liver biopsy will confirm diagnosis.

Treating Complications of Liver Failure

Treating the underlying cause of the cirrhosis is the first step, and in all cases, a healthy diet and avoidance of alcohol are part of the treatment.

Damage to the liver from cirrhosis cannot be reversed, but treatment can stop or slow down further progression and help avoid some of the complications. When alcohol is the cause, abstinence will stop further progression. When cirrhosis is related to hepatitis, treatment with interferons or corticosteroids will be needed. Cirrhosis caused by fatty liver is treated by losing weight. For Wilson's disease, treating the copper buildup with medications removes the copper. When the liver is too far damaged and complications cannot be controlled, a transplant (discussed later in this chapter) is necessary.

Ascites

The most common cause of ascites, or fluid in the peritoneal cavity, is cirrhosis, especially from alcoholism. Chronic hepatitis and hepatic vein obstruction (Budd-Chiari syndrome) also can be a cause. The mechanisms that produce ascites are complex and not completely understood, but two important factors in liver disease are the buildup of bilirubin and high portal vein pressure. These seem to act in concert to alter the fluid exchange across the peritoneal membrane. Circulating blood volume usually is normal or high, yet the kidney behaves as if it were low and avidly retains waste fluids. The kidney itself also may be involved in the process.

Cirrhotic ascites, especially in alcoholics, can become infected without an apparent source. This condition is called spontaneous bacterial peritonitis. Diagnosis may be difficult because the fluid masks any signs of peritonitis. Peritonitis is a medical emergency that needs to be treated immediately.

Symptoms and Diagnosis of Ascites

In small amounts, ascites may produce few symptoms other than abdominal discomfort. Ultrasound and CT can detect smaller amounts of fluid, and a doctor can tell by palpating the abdomen. When the abdomen is tapped with the fingertips, a dull sound is heard, and sometimes there is a visible fluid wave (like a water bed). In advanced cases the stomach is taut and the navel is flat or popping up. Clinical examination usually differentiates ascites from obesity, gaseous distention, pregnancy, or ovarian tumors or other intra-abdominal masses.

Treating Ascites

Ascites is treated with bed rest, diet restrictions, and diuretics, while urinary output and changes in body weight are monitored. Fluid can be withdrawn from the abdomen by paracentesis, a sort of abdominal tap with a long needle. This is done to lower the fluid volume and also to test the fluid. Repeated large-volume paracentesis is a safe and effective means of controlling refractory ascites. Albumin infusion also should be part of the therapy when paracentesis is used. This replaces important proteins that have been lost.

Transjugular intrahepatic portosystemic shunt (TIPS)   This acts like a surgical shunt. It diverts blood away from the congested portal vein into the main venous system. When TIPS is performed for ascites, 60 to 80 percent of patients will have relief. Some of them will no longer need paracentesis. Unlike surgical shunts, TIPS is minimally invasive. It can be done through a small nick in the skin, through which specialized instruments are passed under X-ray guidance. The procedure creates a shunt within the liver itself by using a stent to link the portal vein with a vein draining away from the liver. The stent acts as a scaffold to support the connection between these two veins inside the liver. With the stent in place, the pressure inside the portal veins is relieved.

Portal Hypertension and Esophageal Varices

Blood from the spleen and intestines is normally carried to the liver through the portal vein. This normal flow is slowed by cirrhosis, and thus pressure increases inside the vein. The development of varices (dilated veins within the body) is a serious consequence of portal hypertension.

As blood flow through the portal vein slows down, blood from the spleen and intestines backs up into the blood vessels in the stomach and esophagus. This overload causes those blood vessels to enlarge. They have thin walls and carry high pressure and so are more likely to burst. Rupture causes vomiting of blood and bloody or black, tarry stools. Shock can result when large amounts of blood are lost.

Bleeding must be controlled quickly to avoid shock and death and requires emergency hospitalization. Putting the patient on a ventilator protects the airway and prevents blood from going down into the lungs. Using endoscopic therapy, doctors can directly inject the varices with a sclerosing agent or place a rubber band around the bleeding veins. (This is also used in preventive therapy.) A balloon tamponade also may be used to stop bleeding. A tube is inserted through the nose into the stomach and inflated with air to produce pressure against the bleeding veins.

The transjugular intrahepatic portosystemic shunt (TIPS), described earlier, also can be used to treat this condition. Studies show that 90 percent of patients have relieved symptoms. Medications can be used to slow blood flow. If emergency surgery is needed, shunts that pass blood to the vena cava from the portal vein by a graft or resection of part of the esophagus are two treatment options, but this is risky and the success rate is low. Serious bleeding may require liver transplantation.

Hepatorenal Syndrome

Hepatorenal syndrome is progressive kidney failure from the effects of liver dysfunction. It occurs in up to 10 percent of people hospitalized with liver failure. It may be caused by the accumulated effects of liver damage from cirrhosis or alcoholic hepatitis. It is diagnosed when other causes of kidney failure are ruled out.

Symptoms and Diagnosis of Hepatorenal Syndrome

The most common symptom is decreased urine production. When urine is not eliminated from the body, nitrogen-containing waste products accumulate in the bloodstream. There is a drastic reduction in blood flow to the kidneys, but the kidney structure remains essentially normal. Other symptoms are:

- Decreased urine production
- Dark-colored urine
- Jaundice
- Ascites
- Weight gain
- Change in mental status (dementia, delirium, confusion)
- Damage to the nervous system indicated by abnormal reflexes
- Nausea
- Vomiting

There also may be increased breast tissue, decreased testicular size, lesions on the skin, or other signs of liver failure. Along with the decrease in kidney function, hepatic encephalopathy and other signs of liver failure may be present.

Treatment of Hepatorenal Syndrome

This is directed by improving liver function, if possible, and ensuring that circulating blood volume and cardiac output are adequate. All unnecessary drugs, particularly neomycin, NSAIDs, and diuretics, are stopped. Dialysis may improve symptoms, and medications may improve kidney function. Surgical placement of a shunt from the abdominal spaces to the jugular vein or superior vena cava may reduce ascites and reverse some of the symptoms. The kidneys often will instantly function well if the liver disease is corrected, such as with a liver transplant.

Hepatopulmonary Syndrome

This is a triad of liver disease and arterial and pulmonary vascular dilations. Hepatopulmonary syndrome (HPS) occurs in as many as 19 percent of people with cirrhosis. It is a serious condition that involves lung abnormalities and results in low oxygen levels in the blood. Abnormal widening of the blood vessels in the lungs allows blood to flow through the lungs rapidly. Thus the lungs pick up too little oxygen.

The lungs and liver may be involved simultaneously in several diseases such as AAT deficiency and cystic fibrosis. More than 80 percent of patients have signs and symptoms of liver disease, such as ascites, jaundice, or GI bleeding, but in about 18 percent, the symptoms and signs are related to lung disease. Some studies have shown that the more severe the liver disease, the more severe the HPS, but other studies have not made that connection.

The risk of death is high, about 41 percent within 2½ years of occurrence. The causes are mostly nonrespiratory and include GI bleeding, sepsis, and renal failure. No effective medical treatment exists, and liver transplantation is the therapy of choice.

Hepatic Encephalopathy

When the liver is damaged, it cannot remove toxins from the blood. These toxins accumulate in the blood and eventually the brain. This causes hepatic encephalopathy, also called hepatic coma because complications from liver disorder damage the brain and nervous system. This affects the mental state and personality. People may neglect personal appearance, become forgetful, and change sleep habits.

Hepatic encephalopathy may occur as an acute, potentially reversible disorder or as a chronic, progressive disorder associated with liver disease.

The exact cause of hepatic encephalopathy is unknown, but it occurs when the blood circulation bypasses the liver. When the liver cannot properly metabolize and detoxify substances in the body, toxic substances build up in the bloodstream. One substance particularly toxic to the central nervous system is ammonia, which is produced by the body when proteins are digested but is normally detoxified by the liver. The underlying causes can be fulminant hepatitis, alcoholism, drugs, or liver shock (ischemia).

Acute hepatic encephalopathy may be reversible, but the chronic form is often progressive. Both forms may result in irreversible coma and death, with approximately 80 percent fatality if coma develops.

Treating Hepatic Encephalopathy

Hospitalization is required because this is an acute medical condition and because the brain may swell. Treatment includes life support, controlling the precipitating factors, and removing or neutralizing ammonia and other toxins.

In severe repeated cases, the diet has to be changed to reduce protein in order to reduce ammonia production, but not so much that malnutrition occurs. Lactulose may be given to prevent intestinal bacteria from creating ammonia, and as a laxative to evacuate blood from the intestines. Medications that are metabolized by the liver must be avoided, including sedatives and tranquilizers.

Liver Biopsy, Tumors, Cancer, and Transplantation

The only way to get a sample of liver tissue on which to do a biopsy is through a surgical technique. That's why it's included here. Liver cancer may require surgery to cut away the diseased portion of the liver. When the liver is too damaged to save, another liver can be transplanted if a donor is available. This type of surgery is now done successfully in thousands of people each year.

Liver Biopsy

There are several ways to obtain liver tissue, but all of them are considered minor surgery, so they are done at the hospital. A biopsy would normally be done after blood tests show higher than normal levels of liver enzymes or too much iron or copper. An X-ray or other radiological diagnostic test could suggest a swollen liver. Looking at the liver tissue itself is the best way to find out what's causing the problem.

Before scheduling a biopsy, blood samples will be taken to make sure your blood clots properly. Always mention any medications you take, especially those that affect blood clotting, such as blood thinners. One week before the procedure your doctor will remind you to stop taking aspirin, ibuprofen, and anticoagulants. A fasting period—no food or liquid for the eight hours preceding the procedure—is required.

Percutaneous Biopsy

The most commonly performed liver biopsy is percutaneous. Guided by ultrasound, a needle can be inserted into the liver to extract a small piece of tissue. This is an outpatient procedure. While you lie on your back with your right hand above your head, the surgeon will mark the outline of your liver and inject a local anesthetic to numb the area. Then a small incision will be made in the right side near the rib cage, the biopsy needle inserted, and a sample of liver tissue retrieved. In some cases an ultrasound image of the liver helps guide the needle to a specific spot. You will need to hold your breath and be very still so the needle does not nick the lung or gallbladder, which are close to the liver. You may feel pressure and a dull pain. The entire procedure takes about twenty minutes.

A percutaneous biopsy cannot be performed on someone who is extremely obese, or anyone with hemophilia, or a large amount of ascites (fluid in the abdomen). About 2 percent of patients need to be hospitalized after the biopsy from complications such as pain, hypotension, or bleeding in the abdominal cavity.

Laparoscopic Biopsy

While you are under anesthesia, a laparoscope is placed through an incision in the abdomen to send images of the liver to a monitor, while the doctor uses instruments in the laparoscope to remove tissue samples from one or more parts of the liver. This type of biopsy is done when tissue samples are needed from specific parts of the liver, when cancer is being staged, or if there is a peritoneal infection. It cannot be done with anyone who has severe cardiopulmonary failure, intestinal obstruction, or bacterial peritonitis, or who is morbidly obese.

Transvenous Biopsy

This involves inserting a catheter into a vein in the neck and guiding the catheter to the liver. A biopsy needle is inserted into the catheter and then into the liver. Transvenous biopsy is done with people who have blood-clotting problems or fluid in the abdomen.

After the Biopsy

At home, rest is required for eight to twelve hours. For the next week, while the incision and liver heal, any strenuous exertion is to be avoided. A little soreness will remain at the incision site, and there may be pain in the right shoulder. This is caused by irritation of the diaphragm muscle (pain usually radiates to the shoulder) and should disappear within a few hours or days. Tylenol is prescribed for pain, but aspirin or ibuprofen must be avoided for the first week after surgery, because they decrease blood clotting, which is crucial for healing.

Like any surgery, liver biopsy does have some risks, such as puncture of the lung or gallbladder, infection, bleeding, and pain, but these are rare. It takes a week to ten days to get the results.

Liver Cancer

Overall there are about six thousand new cases of liver cancer each year in the United States. More than 90 percent are associated with the typical risk factors, such as cirrhosis from chronic hepatitis or alcohol abuse. A small number result from cellular variants. Three times more men than women get liver cancer. Primary liver cancer is much less common than metastatic liver cancer, which will be discussed later in this chapter.

Primary liver cancer tumors can be hepatocellular cancers (called hepatomas) or cholangiocarcinomas. Hepatocellular cancers most often occur in livers that are damaged by hepatitis B or C or by alcohol with the development of cirrhosis. This fact influences the treatment options and the outcome because surgery on cirrhotic livers is risky, and removing too much may cause liver failure and death. Also, new and multiple tumors may occur anywhere in the liver, even if others have been adequately treated. Liver cancer may metastasize.

There are four main types of primary liver cancer:

- *Hepatoma.* Also known as hepatocellular carcinoma (HCC), this is the most common type and accounts for 85 percent of all primary liver cancers. It is the fifth most common malignant disease in the world and accounts for more than a million deaths a year. It is one of the most frequent cancers in Asia and Africa. It has increased in the United States because of the increasing incidence of hepatitis C and B. HCC develops from the main liver cells called hepatocytes. It usually occurs in people who have a damaged liver from cirrhosis. It is more likely to develop in men than in women. A subtype of hepatoma called fibrolamellar HCC develops in younger women who do not have cirrhosis. It is usually more successfully treated than the principal type of hepatoma.

- *Cholangiocarcinoma.* This starts in the cells that line the bile duct and accounts for around 12 percent of primary liver cancers. Proximal bile duct cancers are in the upper third of the bile duct, nearer to the gallbladder. Distal bile duct cancers are in the lower third of the bile duct, where it runs through the head of the pancreas. There are different types of cholangiocarcinoma, depending on the appearance of the tumor under the microscope. They can be nodular, sclerosing, papillary, or a mixture of these types—nodular-sclerosing.

- *Angiosarcoma (or hemangiosarcoma).* This is an extremely rare cancer and accounts for only 1 percent of all primary liver cancers. It begins in the blood vessels of the liver and is most often diagnosed in people in their seventies or eighties.

- *Hepatoblastoma.* This is very rare and usually affects children under five years of age. Although liver cancer is rare in children, more boys than girls are affected. It is usually treated with surgery and chemotherapy.

Symptoms and Diagnosis of Liver Cancer

Liver cancer may cause discomfort in the upper right abdomen, pain around the right shoulder blade, and jaundice. A hard lump just below the rib cage on the right side where the liver has swollen is another sign. Ultrasound will detect 85 percent of cases, but CT is currently the preferred test because it shows the necrotic center in most tumors. If a CT is inconclusive, MRI can enhance the diagnosis. An angiogram is done to show the blood supply to the tumor. A percutaneous liver biopsy (see page 184) follows imaging with ultrasound or CT.

Treating Liver Cancer with Surgery

Because the liver can regenerate to its normal size, part of it can be safely removed. This means a local cancer can be cut away, as long as 30 percent of the liver remains in the body to regenerate. In the hands of experienced surgeons, large amounts of the liver can now be removed, improving the prognosis for many people with liver cancer. The five-year survival rate is 20 percent for those who have cirrhotic livers and 35 percent for others.

Cryoablation

This is a technique that freezes the tumor so it dies. Guided by intraoperative ultrasound, a metal tube is placed into the tumor. The tube is cooled to –360 F and an ice ball engulfs the tumor. Later, the dead tumor is reabsorbed by the body.

Radiofrequency Ablation (RFA)

This is a similar process, but it uses heat waves to kill the tumor. Heat is generated through agitation caused by alternating electric current (radiofrequency energy) moving through tissue. Using ultrasound, CT scan, or MRI guidance, a needle electrode is positioned strategically within the area to be treated. The needle is connected to a unique radiofrequency generator, and electrical current is delivered into the tissue. If the procedure is done laparoscopically, it takes about twenty minutes. It can be repeated as necessary.

Liver Transplantation

This may be a viable treatment for small, inoperable liver tumors less than five centimeters in diameter with one nodule, or less than three centimeters in diameter with two or three nodules. Prognosis is about 80 percent for disease-free survival in four years. Adjuvant chemotherapy given after transplantation has shown promising early results in randomized clinical trials. Transplantation is superior to resection for relapse-free survival with large tumors.

Chemotherapy

Systemic chemotherapy has many side effects, and with liver cancer it carries a high risk of the tumors recurring over the next three to four years, so doctors have developed ways to target the chemotherapy.

Hepatic Artery Infusion

This brings the medications through a catheter into the artery that goes to the liver. The catheter can be inserted at the time of liver surgery or in a subsequent operation. This technique produces better tumor response with less toxicity than systemic chemotherapy. A catheter is inserted into the specific artery that supplies blood to the tumor. A chemotherapy drug is then infused, followed by another drug to stop further blood flow to this area. This is generally an outpatient procedure and requires only sedation but not general anesthesia.

Embolization with Chemotherapy

Also called chemoembolization, this not only targets the medications into the tumors but also keeps them there by interrupting the blood supply until the tumor dies. This procedure, using doxorubicin plus mitomycin C, shrinks more than 75 percent of tumors. There are several variations of this treatment.

A team of interventional radiologists, radiation oncologists, and medical oncologists works together to perform chemoembolization or chemoradiation.

Radiation

In general, there is little role for radiation in liver cancer, but when the cancer is in the bile ducts, medical oncologists and radiation oncologists work together to insert tubes into the bile ducts. They deliver iridium 192, a radioactive isotope, through the tubes. Usually this is performed along with traditional radiation and chemotherapy.

Investigational Therapies

Several new treatments are being studied in clinical trials. Adoptive immunotherapy is a way to force the immune system to kill the cancer. Lipiodol is a stable fatty acid from poppy seed oil that contains iodine and works well as a radiocontrast agent. It is selectively taken up by the liver cancer cells. A single dose of this drug after surgery reduced recurrence rate 50 percent after nearly three years. Percutaneous ethanol (alcohol) injection into the tumor may be beneficial. Studies in 1992 showed that survival rates with this treatment were better than with no treatment and equivalent to those of surgery.

Follow-up Care

Tumor size is the most important predictor of survival rates from liver cancer. Small tumors treated with surgery or transplation can be cured. If the tumor is less than 5 centimeters in diameter, there's an 80 percent two-year survival rate. If the tumor is larger than 5 centimeters in diameter, that rate drops to 40 percent. Postsurgical staging also is an important factor. Stage I cancer has a 38 percent five-year survival rate. For Stage II it drops to 35 percent, and Stage III is 17 percent.

Many people who develop liver cancer have such damaged livers that the complications from that have limited their chances of surviving long after cancer. However, many of the treatments extend life for several years with an improved quality of life.

Metastatic Liver Tumors

When tumors from other parts of the body migrate to the liver, it is known as metastatic liver cancer. These cancers are about thirty times more common than primary liver cancer. Colon cancer is the most common, but gastric and pancreatic cancers also lead to liver masses. Hodgkin's disease may involve the liver but usually is not nodular.

Cancers from the lung, stomach, pancreas, and skin must be treated systemically. However, breast tumors or sarcomas can be treated with surgery if they are small in number and not fast-growing in the liver. Neuroendocrine cancer (carcinoid, insulinoma) usually responds to local treatment, too, because it reduces symptoms and survival is long-term.

Treating Metastatic Liver Tumors

Tumors that began in the colon or rectum seem most responsive to treatment (colorectal cancer is discussed in chapter 10). About 25 percent of people with these metastases have cancer that has spread only to the liver, which means local treatment with surgery is likely to succeed. The ideal treatment is to combine surgery with cryoablation or radiofrequency ablation to completely remove and kill all the tumor cells in the liver.

The number of tumors in the liver as well as their size and location will determine whether surgery will help. The surgical approach usually is determined by what the surgeon finds while he or she feels the liver in the operating room and uses the ultrasound machine. Sometimes more tumors are found than predicted by initial CT or MRI scanning.

If the metastasized tumors recur in the liver, repeat operations or ablations often can be performed.

Adjuvant Chemotherapy

Follow-up with systemic chemotherapy is needed to be sure all the tumors in the body are reached. This is done with 5-Fluorouricil (5-FU) or Comptosor (CP-11). Most colon cancer patients with metastasized liver tumors get one or both of these drugs. The chemicals rarely kill the entire tumor, so it is usually combined with other treatments.

Liver Transplantation

Liver transplantation has been performed successfully for forty years. Many people who have had transplants now lead normal lives. At the turn of the twenty-first century, forty-five hundred liver transplants were being carried out each year in the United States. There are about fifteen thousand people on the waiting list, with an average waiting time of a year and a half. More than three thousand people die waiting for transplants.

In adults the most common reason for transplantation is cirrhosis caused by hepatitis or alcohol, autoimmune disease, or fatty liver. Cancer and hereditary liver diseases also lead to transplantation. In children the most common reason is biliary artesia, a condition where bile ducts are missing or damaged. Most people getting liver transplants survive for five years or more.

David Perl, an ultrasound technician at New York Presbyterian Hospital in New York, is still thriving after eleven years with a transplanted liver. At age thirty-four, Perl, married and the father of two sons, was diagnosed with sclerosing cholangitis. After a transplant team stabilized him, Perl waited nine months for a liver. At 2:00 A.M. on the eve of his thirty-fifth birthday, he was called to the hospital, where he was prepped for sixteen hours of surgery. His donor was a forty-two year old man who died of a brain aneurism. After four months, Perl was back at work. After eight months he was going backpacking again. And after three years, his daughter was born. Now, after eleven years, he has a full life.

Transplants can come from several sources. Cadaveric donors account for about 90 percent of transplants. These are whole livers from people who have just died. A living donor who donates the right lobe is common for transplants in both adult and children. The five hundred living donors who do this each year return to work within ten days of surgery. All living donors and donated livers are tested before transplant surgery to be sure the liver is healthy, matches the blood type, and is the right size so it has the best chance of working in its new location.

Because of the shortage of human donors, clinical trials are testing genetically altered (transgenic) pig livers as a temporary bridge to help people with end-stage liver disease. These are used as *ex vivo* (outside the body) until a human donor becomes available. This is done with perfusion, a process similar to dialysis whereby the blood is diverted outside the body through a catheter, passes through the pig liver to remove toxins, then returns to the patient.

Getting On the Waiting List

Names are placed on a national waiting list kept at the United Network for Organ Sharing (UNOS). Blood type, body size, and degree of disease all play a role in when a liver will be received. Currently the sickest people are at the top of the list. During this waiting period, doctors and candidates for transplant work out a plan to keep strong for the surgery and begin learning how to take care of a new liver.

Before the Operation

The social and psychological dynamics of needing a liver transplant also are considered with the medical treatment. For people with liver cancer for whom transplant is the only possible way they will live longer, it has a profound impact. They fear that during the waiting time they will not survive until they get a transplant. They are totally dependent on the medical team. They feel happy when they learn they are about to get the transplant. Then the happiness of getting the transplant may be overshadowed by worry of rejection.

Several medical centers specialize in liver transplantation. The transplant team usually includes a surgeon, liver specialists, nurses, and other health-care professionals. The team will arrange blood tests, X-rays, and other tests that help make the decision about whether a transplant can be carried out safely. Overall health must be considered, such as your heart, lungs, kidneys, immune system, and mental health, to be sure you are strong enough for this surgery.

You cannot have a transplant if:

- Cancer exists in another part of your body
- You have serious heart, lung, or nerve disease
- You are an active alcohol or recreational drug abuser
- You have an active, severe infection
- You cannot follow your doctor's instructions
- You are too young or too old for a hospital's age limit

The Surgery

If the new liver is from a person who has recently died, surgery starts when the new liver arrives at the hospital. If the new liver is from a living donor, both recipient and donor will be in surgery at the same time.

Transplant surgery can take from four to fourteen hours and involves many people. While the surgeon removes the diseased liver, other doctors prepare the new one. The diseased liver is disconnected from the bile ducts and blood vessels before it is removed. The blood that normally flows into the liver will be blocked or sent through a machine to return to the rest of the body. The healthy liver will be put in place and reconnected to bile ducts and blood vessels, and blood will then flow into the new liver.

Preventing Rejection

Recovery in the hospital will take an average of one to three weeks to be sure the new liver is working. Medications to prevent rejection of the new liver and to prevent infection will be given. Doctors will check for bleeding, infections, and rejection. Eating begins again, first with clear liquids, then with solid food as the liver begins to work.

The immune system keeps us healthy by fighting against things that don't belong in our body, such as bacteria and viruses. It is common after a transplant for the immune system to fight against the new liver and try to destroy it. Steroids, cyclosporine, and other immunosuppressant drugs help prevent rejection.

However, with a weakened immune system there is an increased risk of infection, so it is critical to stay away from people who are sick. The drugs also increase blood pressure, damage kidneys, raise cholesterol, and can cause diabetes and osteoporosis. Some steroids cause weight gain. Doctors will monitor these effects and may treat you for complications.

Checking liver enzymes is an important way to monitor any signs of rejection. Rejection can also cause pain, fever, nausea, and jaundice. Sometimes a liver biopsy is needed to be sure the transplanted liver is not being rejected.

The most common problem in liver transplantation is the return of the problem that made the transplant necessary in the first place. Hepatitis C may damage a transplant if the patient was infected before the operation took place. Other problems include blockage of blood vessels to and from the liver, and damage to the bile tubes into the intestine.

About 80 to 90 percent of liver transplants are still working after one year. If the new liver does not work or your body rejects it, doctors will decide whether another transplant is feasible.

After leaving the hospital, frequent visits to the doctor will be necessary to continually monitor the new liver and how it is functioning. A healthy low-fat diet, exercise, and abstinence from alcohol are important for continued success. Most people go back to their normal daily activities, including sex, but getting full strength back will take some time, depending on how sick they were before the transplant. Women must avoid becoming pregnant in the first year after transplantation.

Contact the United Network for Organ Sharing (UNOS) at www .unos.org or by phone at 1-888-894-6361.

Other Conditions of the Liver

Abscesses, cysts, and tumors can affect the liver and sometimes cause serious complications. Pregnant women often have liver problems because of metabolic changes to their bodies, but also because the liver gets pushed by the expanding fetus.

Liver Disease in Pregnancy

The increase in estrogens along with the increased blood volume of pregnancy change the chemical production of the liver, and this induces a mildly cholestatic state. While the changes of pregnancy alter liver biochemistries, normal pregnancy does not significantly affect liver metabolism or function. It does change liver size, however, and a small amount of swelling is common. In the third trimester, the enlarging uterus pushes the liver toward the back.

While changes of pregnancy can create symptoms that mimic liver disease, it is also possible for a pregnant woman to have liver disease, but established chronic disease is unusual. In case it does exist, and depending on the degree of damage to the liver, a pregnant woman may be at risk for hemorrhage from esophageal varices, the most significant complication of cirrhosis in pregnancy. The increased blood volume and flow that are part of normal pregnancy raise the pressure in the esophageal veins. In established cirrhosis this increases the likelihood of bleeding.

When features of liver disease occur during pregnancy, prompt evaluation is essential as some conditions, such as acute fatty liver of pregnancy, rapidly progress to become fatal to both mother and child.

Viral Hepatitis

Having viral hepatitis while pregnant is usually accompanied by malnutrition and poses a significant risk to survival of the fetus. Babies born to mothers with hepatitis B must receive vaccine and medications to control the disease to prevent damage to their liver (see the discussion of hepatitis B in chapter 9).

Gallstones

Elevated estrogen levels increase cholesterol levels in the bile and decrease movement of the gallbladder. Both can lead to gallstones. Estrogen decreases bile acid production, so the cholesterol doesn't get solubilized—(thinned out).

Acute Fatty Liver

Acute fatty liver of pregnancy almost always occurs in the third trimester, with a peak frequency at about thirty-six or thirty-seven weeks' gestation. Sometimes it will become apparent only after delivery. Whenever marked nausea and vomiting develop in the third trimester, this condition should be considered. Suspicion increases if a woman is carrying twins or there are signs of toxemia. Ultrasound and CT scans can detect the increased fat in the liver and help exclude other possibilities. Naturally, it would be dangerous to do a liver biopsy, but it's important to determine that the cause is not due to something else, such as hepatitis. Rapid delivery of the baby may be necessary.

Intrahepatic Cholestasis

Intrahepatic cholestasis of pregnancy accounts for 20 to 25 percent of cases of jaundice during pregnancy. The cause is unknown, but there is a clear genetic predisposition—it is more common in women of Scandinavian or Chilean descent. The cholestatis (failure of bile formation) is an exaggerated response of the liver to the normal increase in estrogens during pregnancy. This, too, happens in the third trimester with the onset of pruritus, itching with no rash.

About half of the women get jaundice, dark urine, and occasionally pale stool. Otherwise women feel well and rarely have nausea, vomiting, or pain. Other than the pruritus, this is a benign condition for the mother, but the cholestasis may increase premature delivery and risk survival of the baby. Delivery should be done as soon as the baby's lungs are developed to prevent increased risk of stillbirth. Treatment is with bile salt binding agents such as cholestyramine. Blood tests and CT scan will not detect this condition, so diagnosis must rule out all other possible causes of symptoms.

Symptoms usually abate within two weeks of delivery. It can recur with subsequent pregnancies and with the use of oral contraceptives and other estrogens.

The HELLP Syndrome

HELLP (hemolysis, elevated liver enzymes, low platelets) usually is associated with pre-eclampsia, a disorder that affects both mother and baby during pregnancy. It is a progressive condition of high blood pressure, swelling, and protein in the urine. It typically occurs during the late second or third trimester. Proper prenatal care is necessary to diagnose and manage this condition. Symptoms include weight gain, headaches, and changes in vision, but some women have few symptoms.

Occasionally HELLP may arise in the absence of either hypertension or proteinuria (too much protein in the urine). Liver complications are similar to those in pre-eclampsia, where the liver is tender and has an abnormal biochemistry. It is critical to distinguish this condition from acute fatty liver, but it may be difficult.

Benign Liver Tumors and Masses

Not all tumors or masses of the liver are cancerous. There are many benign tumors, and new procedures such as freezing (cryoablation) or heating (radiofrequency ablation) have made it easier to treat or remove them without complications. They can be surgically removed or treated with medications. Progress in imaging gives us the chance to find many tumors while they are very small. Having a mass on your liver doesn't always bring symptoms. Many people are surprised when it is discovered because they often feel perfectly normal.

Hemangiomas

Hemangiomas are the most common benign tumors of the liver. They arise from blood vessel tissue, rarely rupture, and can be left alone and followed with periodical ultrasound or CT scan. (They must be distinguished from more serious liver masses.) The only reason to remove them would be if they continue to grow or cause pain.

Several drugs are suspected of promoting the growth of these tumors, including steroid therapy and estrogen therapy. Pregnancy may increase the size of an existing hemangioma.

The reported incidence of hepatic hemangiomas in the United States is about 2 percent. Women, especially those who have had many pregnancies, are affected more often than men. Women also get these tumors at a younger age and have larger tumors. They occur at all ages but are more common in older people.

Most hepatic hemangiomas ar small, and if they present no symptoms are likely to remain that way. They are found with ultrasound, CT scan, and MRI. No treatment is required. However, if symptoms develop and the tumor grows large enough to create a risk of rupture, it may have to be removed surgically.

Focal Nodular Hyperplasia

Focal nodular hyperplasia (FNH) is the second most common tumor of the liver. In the United States, FNH accounts for 8 percent of all primary hepatic tumors. It stems from a process in which all the normal constituents of the liver are present but in an abnormally organized pattern. These tumors are not associated with cancer and often are not treated. If they continue to grow large, or if they are near the surface of the liver where they could rupture and bleed, they need to be removed.

The use of contraceptives may make women vulnerable. Most of these tumors are found incidentally during liver scanning, angiography, CT, or other tests.

Hepatic Adenomas

Hepatic adenomas usually occur in young women and are associated with long-term use of oral contraceptives. There has been a dramatic rise in cases since the advent of oral contraceptive pills in the 1960s. These are large, fleshy tumors that often appear in clusters and sometimes can be detected on clinical examination.

Familial diabetes also is a risk factor. Because they can rupture and cause pain, these adenomas may need to be surgically removed.

Liver Abscess

A liver abscess is a collection of pus in the liver and is usually a result of an intestinal infection (bacterial or parasitic) carried through the blood to the liver. Liver abscess is relatively rare. Biliary tract disease remains the most common source, accounting for 60 percent of cases. The infection is more common in tropical areas where crowded living conditions and poor sanitation exist. Recent travel to a tropical area is a risk factor. Other risk factors include malnutrition, old age, pregnancy, steroid use, cancer, immune system dysfunction, and alcoholism. In the United States, institutionalized people and male homosexuals are known high-risk groups.

Symptoms include fever, pain in the upper right part of the abdomen, malaise, sweating, chills, loss of appetite, jaundice, diarrhea, weight loss, and joint pain. A liver abscess can be diagnosed with ultrasound or CT scan, liver function tests, and blood tests.

It is treated with antibiotics. Rarely the abscess may be drained to relieve some of the abdominal pain. Without treatment the abscess can rupture and spread into the peritoneal cavity and other organs such as the lungs and the area around the heart.

Hepatic Cysts

Hepatic cysts are most common in the right lobe of the liver. Related to polycystic renal disease, the cysts tend to develop in extremely large livers and in people with a protuberant abdomen.

Before the widespread use of abdominal imaging techniques such as ultrasonography and CT scanning, liver cysts were diagnosed only when they grew to an enormous size and became apparent as an abdominal mass or an incidental finding during surgery. The cause of most liver cysts is unknown, but they are believed to be congenital. Polycystic liver disease is congenital and usually associated with kidney disease. People with liver cysts that cause symptoms usually have a dull right upper quadrant pain, abdominal bloating, or early satiety.

No medical therapy has been effective in reducing the size of simple hepatic cysts. Needle aspiration under the guidance of ultrasound or CT is technically simple, but is not done because the cyst grows back nearly all the time.

"Unroofing" the cyst is more effective. This laparoscopic surgical technique excises the portion of the cyst that extends to the surface of the liver. The result is a saucerlike appearance in the remaining cyst so that any fluid secreted from the cells leaks into the peritoneal cavity, where it can be absorbed without any harm.

In cases of polycystic liver disease, the goal is to decompress as much of the cystic liver as possible with a combination of unroofing and fenestration (resection of the involved portion of the liver).

Echinococcal Cysts

These are rare and caused by a parasite, usually from lake water or animal dung. They are cysts within cysts and usually occupy the right lobe of the liver. They can cause obstruction. Hydatid disease is a condition caused by infection with the Echinococcus granulosa. This infection is most often seen in Mediterranean areas, Australia, and South America. The lung, brain, and bone also can be infected. It may cause pain and in some people can cause jaundice, skin rashes, or itching. Treatment involves medication and laparoscopic surgery.

Chapter 10

The Colon and Rectum

THE MAIN FUNCTION OF THE COLON is to concentrate previously digested material by absorbing water and salt before passing it to the rectum, where it is evacuated. Billions of bacteria live in the colon and produce hydrogen, carbon dioxide, hydrogen sulfide, and methane. Mucus secreted by the colon lining contains antibodies that protect the colon from disease.

The colon is connected to the small intestine by a short segment called the cecum. This, along with the colon and rectum, form the entire large intestine, which is approximately four to five feet long. The contents of the colon are propelled through it by coordinated muscular movement (peristalsis). Waste material moves more slowly through the colon than it does through the small intestine, to allow the colon to absorb about two pints of water a day.

The rectum is about 5 inches long and usually is empty except just prior to defecation. The anal canal is just below the rectum and is about $1\frac{1}{2}$ inches long and lined with vertical ridges called anal columns. There are two concentric circular sheets of muscles called the internal and external sphincters, which act like valves and relax during defecation.

The colon and rectum can develop any number of problems—both organic and functional—that can upset the dynamics of this system.

- Inflammatory bowel disease
- Crohn's disease
- Ulcerative colitis
- Irritable bowel syndrome
- Diverticulosis and diverticulitis
- Colon polyps and polyposis syndromes
- Colon cancer
- Anorectal and perianal disorders

Inflammatory Bowel Disease

Inflammatory bowel disease (IBD) refers to Crohn's disease, ulcerative colitis, and a variety of associated conditions. The characteristic finding is inflammation of the lining and wall of the colon. Such inflammation causes the colon to become red and swollen, ulcerate, bleed, and secrete mucus. With Crohn's disease the inflammation extends through the entire wall of the colon and can cause it to thicken and ultimately narrow the passageway. Ulcerative colitis affects only the mucosal lining of the colon wall. Both diseases can remain in remission with periodic acute flare-ups, or become chronic. Chronic ulcerative colitis is known as CUC.

Symptoms for both conditions are similar: diarrhea, abdominal cramping and pain, and rectal bleeding. Abdominal pain of Crohn's disease often is on the lower right side, while ulcerative colitis pain is more common on the left. IBD also can cause fatigue, loss of appetite, weight loss, and loss of body fluids and nutrients. When bleeding is present it can lead to anemia. In some cases joint pain, redness and swelling of the eyes, and skin and liver problems also can occur with IBD. We are not sure why the disease is linked to these problems, but they seem to be mitigated as the IBD is managed. Some people with IBD have only mild symptoms, while others have severe symptoms that may lead to hospital treatment and intravenous feeding (total parenteral nutrition).

The cause of IBD is unknown, but since 1932 there has been strong suspicion that it is based on genetics because the disease does seem to run in families. As many as a third of people with IBD have a relative with the disease. Evidence for a genetic link in IBD also comes from two other observations: prevalence varies according to ethnic background, and risk increases when an identical twin has the disease.

Judy Cho, M.D., a research scientist at the University of Chicago, led a team that made a milestone discovery in the hunt for a genetic link to IBD. In the summer of 2000, the team found that many patients with Crohn's disease have mutations in a gene called NOD-2. If you have one copy of those mutations, your risk of developing Crohn's disease is about two to four times greater than for the general population. If you carry two copies of the NOD-2 mutations, your chance of developing Crohn's disease increases twenty to forty times. Not everyone with the abnormality will get IBD, but genetic testing may help determine the risk.

Changes in the immune system also have been discovered in people with IBD, but we still don't know what causes these changes. Although there is no evidence that stress causes the disease, it is thought to aggravate the symptoms in some people. IBD also is a disease of Western countries but is rare elsewhere in the world. Incidence among whites is about four times that of other races. IBD is observed most commonly in northern Europe and North America. Incidence is higher in Ashkenazi Jews (who have emigrated from northern Europe) than in other groups. A milder and more common form of colonic ailment is irritable bowel syndrome (IBS), which is covered later in this chapter.

IBD most frequently occurs when people are in their late teens, twenties, or thirties. Children and the elderly have been known to have it, but this is less common. When children get this disease, their growth and development are often delayed. The condition affects men and women equally.

Ulcerative colitis can be left-sided, affecting the descending sigmoid colon only, or it can be universal, throughout the length of the colon. When ulcerative colitis is located in the rectum only, it is called proctitis (discussed later in this chapter). Crohn's disease sometimes affects part of the end of the small intestine, the terminal ileum. About 30 percent of people with Crohn's disease have inflammation only in the lower part of the small intestine. This is ileocolitis. But more than half have inflammation in both the ileum and the colon ileocolitis. About 15 percent have it only in the colon, and this is called Crohn's colitis.

Sometimes Crohn's disease affects other parts of the gastrointestinal system. Aphthous ulcers, similar to cold sores, are common, and they can occur in the mouth, esophagus, stomach, and upper small intestine.

Complications of Inflammatory Bowel Disease

Blockage of the intestine is an important and common complication of Crohn's disease. This occurs when the disease thickens the intestine wall with swelling and scar tissue. The hollow passageway (gut lumen) becomes smaller until it finally closes.

A third of people with Crohn's disease get fistulas, which develop when ulcers in the intestine break through the intestine wall to form an abnormal passage between two organs, or from an internal organ to the surface of the body. Fistulas commonly occur around the rectum and anus. They can become infected and form abscesses and sometimes need to be surgically removed. Severe ulcerative colitis could result in perforation of the colon.

The Cancer Risk of Chronic Ulcerative Colitis   About 5 percent of CUC patients will get colorectal cancers, and the longer they have this disease, the greater the risk. CUC patients tend to be younger than the ordinary colon cancer patient at the time of diagnosis. The cumulative probability of developing colorectal carcinoma is 3 percent at fifteen years, 5 percent at twenty years, and 9 percent at twenty-five years. Sixty percent of the people with CUC of the entire colon for more than thirty years will get colon or rectal cancer. Crohn's disease has a lower but real cancer risk. About 2 percent of people with this disease eventually get colon cancer.

Other Types of Inflammatory Bowel Disease

Some rare forms of inflammatory bowel disease include microscopic colitis and clostridium difficile colitis.

Microscopic Colitis

This has two sub-categories: lymphocytic colitis and collagenous colitis. As with Crohn's disease and ulcerative colitis, with which it can co-exist, the cause of microscopic colitis is unknown. Both entities are characterized by chronic nonbloody, watery diarrhea, which can cause between three and twenty bowel movements a day, often accompanied by cramps. Women outnumber men nine to one with collagenous colitis, but there is no gender difference in lymphocytic colitis. The symptoms of both can easily be mistaken for irritable bowel syndrome, but that condition usually begins earlier in life and alternates with constipation. Microscopic colitis usually begins when people are in their sixties or older. Also, it often affects people with autoimmune diseases such as diabetes, celiac disease, rheumatoid arthritis, scleroderma, and CREST.

To confirm diagnosis, a colonoscopy with multiple biopsy specimens throughout the colon is recommended. Collagenous colitis can be distinguished from lymphocytic colitis by the presence of a thickened collagen layer in the lining of the colon.

Dietary modification, such as avoiding coffee and lactose foods, is the standard treatment. Some over-the-counter remedies such as fiber supplements, anti-motility drugs, or bismuth compounds also may help.

Clostridium Difficile Colitis

This often develops after antibiotics are given to hospitalized patients. It causes as many as three million cases of diarrhea and colitis a year and is more common in the elderly. Diarrhea develops during or shortly after starting antibiotics, but 25 to 40 percent may not get symptoms for as many as ten weeks after completing antibiotic therapy. Mild to moderate watery diarrhea, cramping, malaise, anorexia, and fever also are symptoms, along with lower abdominal tenderness and dehydration. The most common antibiotics implicated include cephalosporins, ampicillin, amoxicillin, and clindamycin. Less commonly implicated are the macrolides such as erythromycin, clarithromycin, azithromycin, and other penicillins. Prolonged use of antibiotics, or the use of two or more of them, increases risk of the disease. Even the antibiotics used to treat Clostridium difficile colitis (oral vancomycin or oral metronidazole) have been known to cause the disease.

Diagnosis of Inflammatory Bowel Disease

The symptoms of IBD can resemble other gastrointestinal conditions, such as irritable bowel syndrome, so your doctor will need an extensive history from you. An examination may include blood tests and stool samples. Further testing would possibly include a sigmoidoscopy, colonoscopy, barium enema, CT colonography study of the colon, and/or an upper gastrointestinal series X-ray study of the colon with small-bowel follow-through examination. (You will find details about these procedures in chapter 3.) If the form of IBD known as Crohn's disease is present and is mild, only superficial ulcers will appear on the endoscopic testing. But with deeper ulceration the lining of the colon may look like a cobblestone street and indicate a more chronic disease. The abnormalities may be patchy, with some areas of the colon appearing normal. Your physician may want to endoscope the small intestine as well to see if the ileum is affected.

Treatment Options for Inflammatory Bowel Disease

In recent years there has been a dramatic increase in research and development of new drugs to treat IBD. As a result, there are more treatment options. There is no medical cure for IBD, but there are many drugs that keep it under control. (Ulcerative colitis can be cured by surgically removing the colon, but this is not true for Crohn's disease.)

There is no single ideal therapy for IBD because everyone is unique and drugs affect people differently. If you have Crohn's disease or ulcerative colitis, the first step in treatment is to get the disease under control, and into a place where it can lead to remission so you avoid long-term complications or surgery. The next step is to keep it in remission with medications and nutritional support. Follow your medication program religiously. Medications won't work if you don't take them. Often, people feel okay and figure they don't need to take them, but this puts you at risk for relapse.

Aminosalicylates

This was the first class of drugs that worked with IBD, but it had side effects such as headache, rash, and nausea. Now there are new drugs in this class that don't cause the side effects in 90 percent of the people who take them. They come in pill form, but also can be taken through an enema or suppository. A foam formulation also is ready but is not yet approved by the FDA. In general, aminosalicylate pills, enemas, and suppositories are the first-line therapy for controlling symptoms of active ulcerative colitis and Crohn's disease, as well as for maintaining remission.

Corticosteroids

Prednisone, Medrol, and other drugs in this class also control inflammation. In mild to moderately active disease these drugs in pill form are very effective. However, when the disease is severe, corticosteroids must be delivered intravenously. As many as a third of patients will not respond to corticosteroid treatment. Some become dependent on steroids that cannot be withdrawn without having flare-ups from the disease. Because steroids affect the body's hormone balance they must be withdrawn gradually to avoid serious side effects such as osteoporosis, cataracts, weight gain, diabetes, hypertension, and psychiatric problems. Treatment with these drugs, such as adding calcium and vitamin D to offset bone loss, also involves preventing the side effects.

In 2001 the FDA approved Entocort EC (budesonide), a new class of corticosteroid that is nonsystemic. It is rapidly metabolized and quickly cleared from the bloodstream, so the unpleasant side effects are reduced. This drug is approved for mild to moderate active Crohn's disease involving the small intestine and the first part of the large intestine. The traditional corticosteroids usually are used for those who don't respond to aminosalicylates or who need rapid control of the symptoms.

Antibiotics

Although no infectious agent is associated with IBD, researchers believe that by using antibiotics to reduce the intestinal bacteria and by suppressing the intestine's immune system, they can control IBD. The most commonly used antibiotics are metronidazole (Flagyl) and ciprofloxacin (Cipro). They are used for primary active Crohn's disease but have not proven effective for colitis.

Immunomodulators

Immunosuppressive agents such as azathioprine (Imuran) and 6-mercaptopurine (6-MP, Purinethol) are becoming important tools in treating both active and inactive IBD. These drugs modulate the immune system's role in producing inflammatory symptoms, and are less toxic over the long term than corticosteroids. They are generally used when the disease is not responding to steroids, or is only controlled by unacceptably high doses of steroids, and for patients with frequent flare-ups. Both drugs are available in tablet form and have been in use for twenty years.

Biologic Therapy

Unlike steroids, which broadly effect the immune system and cause serious side effects, biologic agents are engineered to act selectively to restore balance without upsetting other immune functions. The first FDA-approved agent was infliximab (Remicade), for moderate to severe Crohn's disease in people who have not responded to more conventional therapy. The drug is a monoclonal antibody made of human and mouse proteins. It works by blocking the cytokine that intensifies inflammation. People with Crohn's disease have increased amounts of this cytokine in their stool.

Other Drugs

Several other therapies are being studied for their possible role in treating Crohn's disease and ulcerative colitis, including drugs used in organ transplant and omega-3 fatty acid (see page 206). Intravenous cyclosporine A may be effective combined with 6-MP or azathioprine for patients who don't respond to steroids. This may reduce the risk of needing surgery.

Nutritional Support

It's much easier to keep IBD under control than it is to get it under control. Nutritional management is part of your therapy, not because your diet causes the disease, but because the disease can leave you malnourished. Your doctor may order a nutritional assessment to find out if you are consuming enough calories, vitamins, and minerals. If you are not, a liquid supplement may be needed.

Although there is no evidence that what you eat has anything to do with developing ulcerative colitis or Crohn's disease, these conditions naturally have an effect on your digestive system and ultimate health. Paying attention to what you eat can help reduce symptoms and promote healing.

With ulcerative colitis, the small intestine is not affected, so most of the nutrients from your food have already been absorbed by the body before the waste gets to the large intestine. However, in some cases of Crohn's disease, part of the small intestine also is inflamed and cannot process food efficiently. Nutrients are not absorbed by the bloodstream, and as a result you can become malnourished.

There are some new concepts involving nutrition as a way to heal IBD, but these are still experimental. Some studies are under way to see if fish or flaxseed oils in the diet or as supplements can reduce intestinal inflammation. Omega-3 fatty acids found in fish produce a prostaglandin that has anti-inflammatory properties. Also being studied are probiotics—good bacteria that restore the intestinal flora. Live-culture yogurt has shown to be helpful in aiding recovery. Also under study are certain minerals such as selenium and calcium, and vitamins such as folic acid.

In the meantime, it is important to maintain a healthy diet, and keep a diary of any foods or patterns of eating that you think have an effect on symptoms. In this way you can eliminate any foods that you associate with problems. Some people avoid milk because they think they are lactose-intolerant because symptoms are similar to those of IBD. Keep in mind, however, that some of those foods may be necessary for certain vitamins and nutrients. By keeping the diary, you can get some idea if you need to take vitamin supplements.

It's also important to drink enough water. Chronic diarrhea puts you at risk for dehydration. Some people with IBD are at increased risk of kidney stones because of dehydration.

People with Crohn's disease often lose their appetite and feel nauseous. This makes them avoid eating. However, when symptoms flare, the body needs more energy to cope—and you need to eat to create energy. Medications also are more effective if you've got good nutritional status. In children, poor nutrition will lead to poor growth. In women and girls who do not maintain a healthy weight, the hormonal balance is upset and results in menstrual irregularities.

Take calcium and vitamin D supplements to avoid bone loss from malnutrition or corticosteroids that interfere with the absorption of calcium, accelerate the breakdown of bone, and slow the process of new bone formation. Ask your doctor about this. Avoid pain relievers and other medications that irritate the intestinal lining. These include aspirin and nonsteroidal anti-inflammatory drugs (NSAIDs) such as Advil and Motrin.

Ways to Reduce Cramping after Eating

While medication should keep your condition under control during flare-ups, there are other ways you can help reduce abdominal distress:

- Eat smaller meals more frequently.
- Cut down on the amount of fried or greasy foods; fat is difficult to absorb.
- Eliminate certain types of high-fiber foods such as nuts, popcorn, and seeds.
- Consider a special liquid diet or low-fiber residue diet to help reduce symptoms.

Enteral Nutrition

People with IBD, especially those with Crohn's disease, may need nutritional support by delivering a nutrient-rich liquid formula directly into the stomach or small bowel. This is known as enteral nutrition and is done overnight while the patient sleeps. A feeding tube called a nasogastric (NG) tube brings the formula through the nose into the stomach. These feedings also can be given through a gastrostomy tube (G tube) via a surgically or endoscopically created opening in the abdominal wall leading directly to the stomach. This can be done by the patient alone or with the assistance of a home nurse.

Total parenteral nutrition (TPN) is delivered through a catheter into a large blood vessel, usually in the chest. This is the least desirable method because it is more expensive and requires more specialized training. The good part is that it bypasses the intestine and allows it to rest.

Surgery for Crohn's Disease

Surgery cannot cure Crohn's disease, but there are times when it may be necessary:

- when the disease is long-lasting and medication does not control it
- when there's a lot of bleeding
- when ulceration has made a hole in the intestinal wall
- when strictures have caused obstruction

About 75 percent of people with Crohn's disease will need surgery at some point. Surgery removes the diseased segment of the intestine in one of two ways:

Strictureplasty

This is the most common surgical procedure for Crohn's disease. A small segment of intestine that has narrowed because of scarring is widened. This opens up the passageway so intestinal contents can move freely.

Resection

This removes a diseased segment and rejoins the two healthy ends. Different types of resection depend on what part of the intestine is removed. When all of the colon is removed and the small intestine is joined to the rectum, it is a total colectomy. If the rectum also is removed it is a proctocolectomy.

Surgery for Ulcerative Colitis

About 25 to 40 percent of people with ulcerative colitis will need surgery. Some will need it because of emergencies such as perforation of the colon wall, massive bleeding, or toxic megacolon—when the muscle wall dilates and gases build up inside the colon. Some people choose surgery, however, because they have chronic severe symptoms or medical therapy does not help—or because they want to reduce their risk of colon cancer.

The procedure most often recommended is the proctocolectomy—removal of the colon and rectum. Today this surgery can be done in a way that avoids the need for an external colostomy appliance by reconstructing part of the small intestine into a pouch that serves as a rectum. Surgery often is done in two stages (but may be done in one). First, the colon and rectum are removed up to the level of the anal muscles. Then the ileum, the very end of the small intestine, is made into a reservoir, pulled down to the anus, and connected with sutures or staples. To let the pouch heal, a temporary loop prevents stool from passing to the new pouch. A temporary ileostomy allows waste matter to leave the body through a stoma in the abdomen and collect in an external appliance. About two months later, in another surgery, the ileostomy is closed and the external appliance is no longer needed.

After this restorative surgery, fecal matter is eliminated normally, but stool is softer and must be eliminated four to six times a day because it no longer has the same kind of storage capacity.

Side Effects of Surgery

Small-bowel obstruction, which can cause pain and vomiting, or pouchitis, an inflammation of the internal pouch, can occur in some people after surgery. The obstruction usually needs to be removed with more surgery. Symptoms of pouchitis can be mild or severe and usually include diarrhea, crampy abdominal pain, and sometimes fever and joint pain. Antibiotics can be used for several weeks to manage the condition. About 30 percent of people with the pouch develop pouchitis.

A more serious complication is pouch failure, which means reversion to a permanent ileostomy. (It is extremely important that anyone considering this surgery consult a surgeon with extensive experience in the procedure.) Ileostomy brings the small bowel through the abdominal wall, allowing intestinal waste to drain through the stoma. The site of the ileostomy is usually just below the belt line on the right side of the abdomen.

Before this surgery it is a good idea to discuss it with your doctors and also with "ostomates," people who have been living with this device and can help you understand how it will affect your lifestyle. While the ileostomy allows for a long, productive life, it is difficult in the beginning to cope with it emotionally. Support from family and physicians is critical. There are local chapters of the Crohn's and Colitis Foundation of America, and similar organizations, where you can find help (see the appendix).

Living with Inflammatory Bowel Disease

Although IBD is a chronic disease, most people have a normal life during periods of remission. Learning to prevent relapse is part of the treatment plan. If you have chronic and continuing symptoms, you need to know your body and how IBD affects you. The more you learn about caring for it yourself, the more control you can exert. It's important to develop a support system that works for you among family and friends—and outside support groups through organizations dedicated to people with the disease.

Guarding against Colon Cancer

Anyone with CUC should have an annual surveillance colonoscopy. In addition, he or she should have multiple biopsies of the colonic mucosa beginning seven years after the onset of universal colitis and fifteen years after the onset of left-sided colitis. The biopsy specimens should be examined under the microscope by pathologists for the presence of precancerous changes called dysplasia. Dysplasia is rated by a grading system as being either absent, low-grade, moderate-grade, or high-grade. When high-grade dysplasia is found, a total proctocolectomy—the removal of the entire colon and rectum—is usually called for.

Pregnancy and IBD

In the past, women with IBD were advised not to get pregnant, but today with better medical management that has changed. If women are supervised by qualified doctors, they should be able to have a healthy pregnancy and baby. Family planning is important because it is not wise to get pregnant during a flare-up or while on certain medications. For example, sulfasalazine may cause temporary infertility in about 60 percent of men. The sulfa component in the drug can alter sperm, but this effect is reversed within two months of stopping the drug. If an unplanned pregnancy occurs during a severe flare-up of IBD, the disease needs to be treated aggressively to achieve a remission.

Some IBD medications are best avoided during pregnancy, but others are considered safe for mother and fetus. The FDA has a classification system for the use of medications during pregnancy. Drugs considered safe to use during pregnancy include sulfasalazine, various forms of mesalamine, and corticosteroids. In the case of serious flare-ups, the immunosuppressive drugs may be recommended with caution. However, there are two immunosuppressive drugs that do have an effect on the fetus—methotrexate and thalidomide. These need to be avoided.

Irritable Bowel Syndrome

Recent advances in treating irritable bowel syndrome (IBS) have helped stem the belief that it is psychosomatic and that nothing much can be done about it. While it is not a disease, it is a very real functional syndrome that involves many of the body's physical and mental systems.

In the past nobody wanted to talk about this condition, which interferes with everyday lives and causes much pain and embarrassment—and stress. But now it is out of the closet and new studies have revealed how underreported it is. According to the National Institutes of Health, one in five— or thirty-five million—Americans has IBS. About two-thirds are women.

Irritable bowel syndrome is a bit like having an unruly child. You never know when it is going to act up. At work, dining out, or traveling, people with this syndrome can suddenly be stricken with diarrhea or doubled over in pain. IBS usually begins in early adulthood with a change in frequency or consistency of bowel movements. At least 25 percent of the time diarrhea or constipation occurs. While it causes a great deal of discomfort and stress, IBS does not permanently damage the colon, nor does it lead to other, more serious diseases.

Here's how it works. After a meal the stomach is distended and releases various gastrointestinal hormones. This activates the nerves in the colon, which in turn stimulate the muscle of the colon wall. This gastrocolic reflex can be exaggerated in people with IBS who may feel a need to rush to the toilet with cramps and diarrhea even before a meal is over.

Regular colon contractions move the contents of digested food back and forth slowly while moving it toward the rectum. During this passage the water and nutrients are being absorbed into the body, leaving the remainder—stool—to be eliminated. These contractions occur several times a day, sometimes resulting in a bowel movement and sometimes resulting in problems. If the muscle action of the colon, the pelvis, and the sphincters are not coordinated, the result is pain, constipation, or diarrhea.

The genesis of IBS is not yet well understood, but at least four systems of the body are involved in its causes and therefore in its treatment:

- *Physiological:* the autonomic nervous system (ANS), neuro-endocrine, and pain sensation
- *Emotional:* anxiety and depression are clearly brought on by the discomfort and fear the condition causes
- *Cognitive:* how the mind translates the condition into behavior and coping styles
- *Behavioral:* how reaction to environmental stresses contributes

Like the heart and lungs, the colon is controlled by the autonomic nervous system (ANS). This is the unconscious part of your nervous system. It tells your colon when to contract and move the contents of your digestive system forward, toward elimination. Because the colon has this connection to the brain, it is easily affected by stress and emotions. When you are frightened, your heart beats faster. The colon responds to stress by contracting too much or too little. Some people's colons are more sensitive than others. And the sensitive colon also responds strongly to stimulation from foods.

Although IBS is not a disease itself, it is associated with some diseases or conditions such as depression, fibromyalgia, chronic fatigue syndrome, abnormal eating behavior, chronic stress, migraines, personality and anxiety disorders, physical and sexual abuse, and sleep disturbance. With some people, IBS can be part of a more global gastrointestinal problem such as reflux disease.

A study released in 2000 claims that IBS may be caused by too much bacteria in the small intestine. The study found that 78 percent of the IBS patients had bacterial overgrowth in the small intestine (see chapter 6). The significance of this finding remains to be determined.

Women Are More Vulnerable

We don't know why women are so much more vulnerable to IBS, but it's thought that there may be some aggravation from the reproductive hormones because many women report worse attacks of IBS during menstrual periods. The pain and symptoms of IBS also can be confused with the pain of endometriosis or ovarian pain. This is why women should have a gynecological examination to get a proper diagnosis of IBS. Victims of physical and sexual abuse more often than others have IBS. This, too, may be a factor in why it is more common in women.

The Society for Women's Health Research did a study recently of the unmet needs of women with IBS. It describes why IBS often goes unrecognized and untreated, the impact on women's lives, and the need for better communication between women and their doctors. For more information, check the society's Web site at www.womens-health.org.

Symptoms of Irritable Bowel Syndrome

Most people can eventually learn to control their symptoms with medication, diet, exercise, and stress management. However, many people with IBS suffer so often that it interferes with their lives. Some fear social events, travel, or even their jobs, because they don't know when the next attack will occur. Will they be able to get to a bathroom in time if diarrhea strikes? Will they be embarrassed by an outbreak of bloating and gas? Or will they suddenly be doubled over in severe pain?

Crampy, abdominal pain is a common symptom of IBS. Alternating constipation and diarrhea also are common symptoms, but one usually predominates. Constipation is more common throughout the course, but diarrhea is more common at the outset. About 25 to 50 percent of people also suffer nausea, vomiting, and/or heartburn.

Some people say their pain stops after moving their bowels, while others feel pain with more frequent bowel movements. Others feel that their movement was incomplete and feel the need to go again. This is called tenesmus. (This also may be a symptom of a tumor or distal colitis.)

Diagnosis of Irritable Bowel Syndrome

The only way to accurately diagnose IBS is to first rule out all other possibilities. Many other gastrointestinal conditions, and even other diseases, have similar symptoms. A medical history and physical examination are critical for diagnosis. An abdominal X-ray can check for fecal impaction or gaseous distension. A stool test must be done to determine if there is any blood present. Although blood is not a symptom of IBS, its presence should prompt a thorough evaluation, because IBS symptoms can be mistaken for many other conditions, including:

- Cancer (particularly ovarian and endometrial)
- Inflammatory bowel disease (IBD)
- Poor blood flow to the intestines (intestinal ischemia)
- Chronic constipation syndromes from poor diet or drugs
- Chronic diarrheas from infectious disease, malabsorption, drugs, or bacterial overgrowth
- Lactase deficiency
- Gynecologic disorders, especially endometriosis, gynecological cysts, and cancer
- Fear of cancer

Treating Irritable Bowel Syndrome

There is no cure for IBS, but there are many new ways to keep in under control. You need to maintain a positive attitude to manage a lifetime condition effectively, however. The emotional aspect of the condition is particularly important, and you need to know that your doctor acknowledges your pain and discomfort. Reassurance from your doctor is critical, and he or she needs to educate you about your condition rather than simply give you a prescription. The doctor may have to devote considerable time for patient counseling, both in the office and on the phone.

Discuss treatment with your doctor because there are many issues to consider, and no two cases are alike. There are four variations of IBS, and symptoms and treatment depend on which variation you have, along with psychological support:

- Pain is predominant.
- Constipation is predominant (cIBS).

- Diarrhea is predominant (dIBS).
- Constipation alternates with diarrhea (mixed or mIBS).

Treatment plans may include prescription drugs to control colon muscle spasms, drugs that slow the movement of food through the digestive tract, tranquilizers and antidepressants, as well as counseling to overcome the anxiety that often accompanies the condition. But the balance is tricky. Medications to treat diarrhea, if taken for too long, can cause constipation, and medications to treat constipation can cause diarrhea. Drugs affect everybody differently, and what works for one may not be as effective for someone else. You and your doctor must set particular goals to develop an initial treatment strategy that focuses on a major symptom such as pain, diarrhea, or constipation.

After several visits with a physician and an evaluation that included thorough blood tests and a colonoscopy, it was concluded that Paula suffered from constipation predominant irritable bowel syndrome. A meeting and follow-up with a dietician were arranged, and she was instructed regarding a high-fiber diet, including fruits, vegetables, and bran cereal. Although some improvement was noted initially, stool softeners and psyllium products were soon added. Finally, she was offered a course of tegaserod (Zelnorm), which improved her bowel pattern and dramatically lessened her symptoms.

When Pain Is Predominant

Diet

Here's where a daily diary of what you eat and when your symptoms occur will come in handy. With your doctor you can figure out if certain foods are triggers to your IBS. Or perhaps it's the amount of food or the conditions in which you are eating. Certain foods are known to trigger IBS. These include chocolate, alcohol, and milk. Caffeine can cause diarrhea, while beans, cabbage, and some fruits cause gas and cramps. Fatty foods and large meals can aggravate IBS. However, not everyone is affected by particular foods, so diet change is not for everyone.

Medication

Nonsteroidal anti-inflammatory drugs (NSAIDs) such as aspirin may relieve moderate pain. If you need stronger pain relief, your doctor may prescribe an analgesic such as tramadol (Ultram).

Tegaserod (Zelnorm) increases the movement of the GI tract and reduces the sensation of pain. This is taken before meals. The main side effect is diarrhea and possibly an increase in gallstones and ovarian cysts. Recently patients have been cautioned about developing ischemic colitis while using Zelnorm. They develop bloody diarrhea, rectal bleeding, or new or worsening abdominal pain. Several other prokinetic agents are available, but they are not appropriate for all patients.

Antispasmodic agents may relieve lower abdominal pain but do not modify the condition. Bentyl (dicyclomine) and other antispasmodics can cause grogginess, dry mouth, difficulty urinating, and a fast heart rate.

Kappa-opiate receptor agonists for pain control are in development. Fedotozine has been tried as a visceral analgesic in various clinical trials, with conflicting results. In humans fedotozine decreases the perception of gut distension both in physiological and pathological conditions. Six-week treatments with the drug relieved abdominal pain.

When Diarrhea Is Predominant

Over-the-counter remedies for diarrhea, such as Imodium, can help some people some of the time. However, drugs taken for a long time to combat diarrhea can lead to constipation.

Diphenoxylate (Lomotil) and cholestyramine (Questran and Questran Light) are effective for those who have high cholesterol, a condition that needs to be controlled through diet and medication. The medications are effective only if diet and exercise are followed. A side effect of these drugs may be constipation.

Alosetron (Lotronex) was reapproved by the FDA in 2002 for women with severe IBS who have not responded to conventional therapy. However, it should be used with extreme caution because of side effects such as decreased blood flow to the colon or severe constipation. This drug was originally pulled from the market because of concerns about constipation and ischemic colitis. More than 160 people were hospitalized, and 6 deaths occurred. One woman was left mostly paralyzed and unable to breathe on her own after a burst colon attributed to alosetron caused a brain-damaging infection. Ischemic colitis occurs when the blood flow to the large intestine is reduced or eliminated. This happened to 1 in 700 patients treated. The incidence of life-threatening side effects of alosetron is extremely high for a drug that treats an illness that is not life-threatening. Some patients with IBS find that alosetron is unique in providing relief. They accept the associated risks by signing a patient-doctor agreement provided by the FDA.

When Constipation Is Predominant

Diet

Add more fiber such as wheat or oat bran or psyllium to your diet. Fruit and vegetables should be eaten every day. Sometimes fiber supplements may be needed. Here are some foods high in fiber:

- Kidney, pinto, and lima beans
- Green peas
- All-Bran, Bran Flakes, Shredded Wheat
- Sweet and white potatoes
- Brown rice
- Whole wheat bread
- Popcorn
- Corn, carrots, Brussels sprouts, zucchini
- Apricots, prunes, pears, grapefruit, orange, banana

Medication

Occasional osmotic laxatives, such as lactulose or polyethylene glycol, may alleviate constipation, but this is not a good idea for the long term. Osmotic laxatives work by retaining fluid in the bowel by osmosis or by changing the pattern of water distribution in the feces. Over time harsh laxatives such as senna and cassava can lead to a flaccid colon that doesn't function properly. Stimulant laxatives that alter peristalsis include phenolphthalein and bisacodyl.

Tegaserod (Zelnorm) was approved by the FDA in 2002 for treating women initially for four to six weeks. This medication activates receptors that normalize the movement of waste through the intestines to facilitate normal bowel movements. In clinical studies of twenty-five hundred women, participants reported relief from pain, discomfort, bloating, and constipation. It also improved their sense of well-being. Side effects may include headache and diarrhea, but most in the study said that happened only once in the first week and then resolved. This prescription drug is taken twice a day on an empty stomach. The safety and effectiveness of this drug in men have not yet been established. And if you have diarrhea, you should not use this drug.

Managing Stress

Stress is a condition of feeling out of control, but it affects everybody differently. Some feel stressed at minor everyday challenges, while others seem to thrive on this type of stress. Feeling mentally or emotionally tense, angry, or overwhelmed is stressful. Because the colon is in tune with your nervous system and brain, the colon can alter its normal contractions at stressful times. Like a vicious circle, the anxiety you suffer from having IBS creates more stress.

Stress plays a large role in acute attacks, and it also has a residual action in the body. Taut muscles set up a chain reaction through the gut. An attack may not occur until several hours after the stress has passed. This is why some people don't always see the connection. Keeping a daily diary can help identify particular stressors in your life.

Getting the upper hand over stress in your life will help you keep IBS under control. Stress management is an important part of treatment. There are various ways of doing this, through exercise, Yoga, and meditation. Ask your doctor for information, and look for stress management courses and self-help groups in your area.

Medication

Tricyclic antidepressants such as Amitril, Elavil, Tofranil, Sinequan, and Desyrel are mild to moderately constipating, but they are good for chronic pain and anxiety. Antidepressants increased response rates more than four times for patients with IBS. The serotonin receptor type-3 antagonist Lotronex has been approved only for women with dIBS, but this agent has been linked with colonic ischemia and severe constipation (see page 215). Benzodiazapines such as Xanax, Valium, and Librium provide short-term anxiety therapy but may worsen constipation. They also can be habit-forming.

Complementary Therapy

A controlled study published in the Journal of the American Medical Association showed that some Chinese herbal formulations appeared to improve symptoms for some patients. However, there is no good way to tell if an herbalist is legitimate or not. Most would not stand up to scientific scrutiny.

Biofeedback, as well as behavioral and psychological therapy, help many people. Biofeedback is a system of education and treatment based on monitoring biological signals produced by the body. Electronic instruments monitor the body's physiology and display the information back on a video screen. This increases awareness of your body's activity and makes it possible for you to control some unconscious systems such as breathing, muscle contraction, and relaxation. Biofeedback has been used for IBS, but there is no proof that it works.

Exercise

Regular exercise such as walking is a great way to work off stress, and it is known to reduce symptoms of IBS. This is also good in general for the colon because it brings more oxygen to the colon and stimulates movement.

What to Know about Diet

Eating carefully and well help many people cope with IBS. The first step is to keep a daily journal and write down everything you eat—along with the circumstances. For example, if you gulp down lunch while working on a deadline project with coworkers, you may put a strain on your sensitive gastrointestinal system. Do you drink ten cups of coffee a day? Do you lunch on cheeseburgers and fries? Excessive drinking of coffee (with caffeine) and alcohol probably contribute to IBS, although it has not been proven. Tobacco wreaks havoc on the digestive tract. It is unhealthy and may increase the amount of gas in the gut. Record all the symptoms and fluctuations of your IBS. After a few weeks you may begin to see patterns that relate to the food you are eating, or activities before or after eating and your symptoms. Some people, even those not known to be lactose-intolerant, may see symptoms after eating or drinking dairy products.

Adding more fiber to your diet is helpful if you are constipated, but it won't do anything to stop diarrhea. High-fiber diets can, however, keep the colon a bit distended because of their bulk, and this can help prevent spasms. Fiber, in some forms, also can keep water in the stool and prevent it from getting too hard to pass. The downside is that high-fiber diets can cause gas and bloating, but in general this goes away when your body adapts to the change. Add these foods gradually to prevent bloating and gas.

Eating smaller portions may help symptoms.

Drinking lots of plain water is important no matter what condition you are in. But it is especially helpful if you have IBS. Drink six to eight glassfuls a day. And don't confuse other liquids with water. Caffeinated drinks such as coffee, tea, or cola, while made with water, actually dehydrate you.

Diverticulosis and Diverticulitis

When a pouch balloons outward from the wall of the colon, it forms what is called a diverticulum. When there is more than one, these herniations are called diverticula. And the condition of having one or more is diverticulosis.

We don't know the exact cause, but diets low in fiber and low physical activity are strongly associated with the development of diverticula because both lead to constipation. This forces the muscles to strain to move stool, thus increasing pressure in the colon. The excess pressure can cause weak spots in the colon to bulge out and become diverticula.

About half of all Americans sixty to eighty, and almost everyone over eighty, have diverticulosis. Many of them don't know it and never have symptoms or discomfort other than mild pain in the lower left abdomen, the site of the descending and sigmoid colon. Right-sided diverticula are uncommon.

The connection between a low-fiber diet and diverticular disease was first noticed in the United States in the early 1900s, when commercially processed foods became widely available here and in other developed countries, especially England and Australia. The disease is rare in Asia and Africa, where people eat high-fiber vegetable diets. Fiber is the part of grains, fruits, and vegetables that the body cannot digest. Some fiber dissolves easily in water (soluble fiber such as oatmeal) and takes on a soft, jellylike texture in the intestines. Some fiber passes almost unchanged through the intestines (insoluble fiber such as raw vegetables). Both types help make stools softer and easy to pass, thus preventing constipation. Physical activity also aids digestion and keeps the colon contents moving so that fecal matter doesn't get stalled and fester in the pouches. If that happens, infection and inflammation develop. This is called diverticulitis, and it can lead to peritonitis, a serious infection of the abdominal cavity. About 10 to 25 percent of people with diverticulosis get diverticulitis.

Diverticulosis

Most people with diverticulosis don't know they have it. They have no symptoms or discomfort. When they do have symptoms, it is often associated with constipation, pain, tenesmus (the feeling of incomplete bowel movements), and sometimes bleeding from the rectum. It is rare for diverticula to bleed, but when they do, it is because a small blood vessel in a pouch weakens and finally bursts. It can be severe or stop by itself and need no treatment, but always see your doctor any time you notice blood in the stool. Other than hemorrhoids, diverticulosis is the most common cause of bleeding from the lower GI tract.

Diverticula are often discovered incidentally during diagnostic tests, such as a colonoscopy or sigmoidoscopy. And if it causes no discomfort, then nothing needs to be done about it. A high-fiber diet and mild pain medications will help relieve symptoms in most cases.

Diverticulitis

Diverticulitis, on the other hand, is a much more serious condition and consists of at least microperforations in the diverticula. This means the pouch has a tiny hole and potentially can leak contents of the colon into the abdominal cavity. Perforations develop from constant straining to move stool through the colon. Sometimes a pouch can rupture and lead to fecal contamination of the peritoneum, the membrane surrounding the abdominal cavity.

A rupture can develop from an abscess, an infected diverticulum with pus that may swell and destroy colon tissue. If the abscess is small and remains in the colon it may clear up after treatment with antibiotics. If it does not clear up, it needs to be drained. A large abscess can become a serious problem if the infection leaks out and contaminates the area outside the colon. Peritonitis requires immediate surgery to clean the abdominal cavity and remove the damaged part of the colon. Without surgery, peritonitis can be fatal.

Another complication of diverticulitis is a fistula, an abnormal connection of tissue between two organs. When damaged tissue comes into contact with another organ it may stick to it. If it heals that way, a fistula forms. When infections from diverticulitis spread outside the colon, the colon's tissue may stick to the nearby bladder, small intestine, or skin. The most common type of fistula forms between the colon and the bladder and affects men more than women. A severe, long-lasting infection of the urinary tract can result, and surgery is needed to remove the fistula and the affected part of the colon.

The scarring caused by infected diverticula may cause partial or total blockage of the large intestine. When this intestinal obstruction happens, the colon is unable to move bowel contents normally and emergency surgery is necessary. Partial blockage is not an emergency, so the surgery to correct it can be planned.

Lillian was seventy, and after twelve hours of pain in her lower abdomen with nausea, constipation, and low-grade fever as well as loss of appetite, she came to see her doctor. She said that six hours before her symptoms began she shared a large canister of popcorn with her husband while at the movies. A year earlier, in a routine colonoscopy, Lillian was told she had diverticulosis in her sigmoid colon. Now, blood work showed that Lillian had an infection, and a CT scan revealed thickening of the colon wall surrounded by "dirty fat" that is typical of diverticulitis. She was treated with three days of a liquid diet and gradually reintroduced to solid food. Ten days of antibiotics helped relieve the symptoms.

Symptoms and Diagnosis of Diverticulitis

Abdominal pain is present in nearly all cases of diverticulitis and emanates from the lower left side. Right-sided diverticulitis is rare. The pain also may be felt in the pubic area in women and in the scrotum or penis in men.

If infection is present, fever, nausea, vomiting, chills, cramping, and constipation also may occur. The severity depends on the infection and complications such as perforations, tears, or intestinal obstruction. Tachycardia, hypotension, and sepsis syndrome may occur as the disease progresses.

A CT scan is the best diagnostic test to detect diverticulitis. An air contrast barium enema (with colonoscopy a close second) is the best way to detect diverticulosis but it is not done in the presence of diverticulitis. An ordinary X-ray also may indicate the presence of air in the abdominal cavity, which usually means there is a perforation.

A digital rectal exam can detect tenderness, blockage, or blood. Blood tests can detect infection, electrolyte imbalances, dehydration, and other problems common to the disease.

Diverticulitis progresses in four stages:

- Stage I: small, confined pericolic abscesses, mild symptoms
- Stage II: larger pericolic abscesses, classic symptoms (localized)
- Stage III: generalized peritonitis is present
- Stage IV: fecal contamination of peritoneal cavity

Treating Diverticulitis

The goal of treatment for diverticulitis is to clear up the infection with antibiotics, rest the colon, and prevent complications. A liquid diet for seven to ten days is part of treatment for mild diverticulitis. Pain-relieving medications must be used with great care so they don't mask worsening pain or increase constipation and the risk of perforation. In more severe cases, all eating and drinking must stop, and nutrients and painkillers are administered intravenously while in the hospital.

Morphine may cause colonic spasm, so the drug of choice for pain is Demerol. Antibiotics are given intravenously.

When a large abscess is present, it may need to be drained. A radiologist does this under X-ray guidance by inserting a small needle through the skin of the abdomen and draining the fluid through a catheter. This procedure is called percutaneous catheter drainage. Sometimes surgery is needed to clean the abscess and, if necessary, remove part of the colon. Usually this is done in the hospital.

Surgery

Up to 20 percent of people with moderate diverticulitis will need surgical intervention. Single-stage procedures are now often possible. This is a way to resect the involved portion of the colon and do the anastomosis in one operation, as opposed to two or three. If attacks are severe and frequent, surgery may be needed to remove the diseased part of the colon and rejoin the remaining sections. Sometimes this is done if a fistula or blockage is evident. Nowadays this can often be done successfully using a keyhole approach, or laparoscopy.

Emergency surgery requires two operations. The first is to clear away infection or blockage and remove the diseased colon section. Because of the infection or obstruction, it is not possible to rejoin the separate parts of the colon at the same time. A temporary stoma will be created so a colostomy bag can be used. Months later a second operation will rejoin the sections of colon, and normal functions return.

Preventing Diverticulitis

The recurrence rate for diverticulitis is about 25 percent, so it's a good idea to prevent its return by sticking with a low-fat, high-fiber diet, but avoid nuts, seeds, and popcorn. Stool softeners (such as Colace) may be useful. Regular exercise must be part of the daily routine.

Refer to the list of high-fiber foods earlier in this chapter.

Colon Polyps and Polyposis Syndromes

A polyp is a new growth of epithelial tissue that serves no purpose. Although polyps of the colon might contain cancer, the word *polyp* usually refers to a benign condition. This kind of growth can occur in the inner lining of the colon when the cells in the mucous membrane—epithelial cells—fail to adhere to their normal routine. This abnormal growth can be caused by genetic programming or by years of wear and tear on the colon. Polyps can grow inside the colon for years without being noticed. Benign polyps are always removed to make sure they are benign and because it is believed that if they stay in the colon long enough, they might become cancerous.

Again, think of the colon and rectum as a long, hollow tube, the inner lining of which is called the mucosa. Polyps and cancers arise from this mucosal lining. A polyp is a protrusion into the gut lumen (the passageway inside of the colon) of a small amount of mucosal tissue. When discovered by barium enema X-ray, colonoscopy, sigmoidoscopy, or during surgery, polyps always are measured by their greatest dimension in millimeters (25.4 millimeters = 1 inch).

Polyps sometimes are further described as sessile or pedunculated, depending on their shape. Sessile polyps have a broad base and often are only slightly raised above the mucosa, whereas pedunculated polyps are attached to the mucosa by a narrow stalk.

When removed and examined after proper processing and staining under a microscope by pathologists, polyps can be further classified by the appearance of their cells and their architecture as adenomatous, hamartomatous, hyperplastic, or inflammatory. These last three are not considered precancerous. Most authorities believe it is the adenomatous polyp that is precancerous, through a mechanism known as the adenoma-carcinoma sequence. Adenomatous polyps can be further subclassified by their histologic appearance into tubular, villous, or tubulovillous types.

More than 95 percent of cancers of the colon are thought to originate in a polyp, and the risk of an adenomatous polyp of the colon or rectum containing cancer appears to be, in part, directly dependent on its size. For polyps less than 1 centimeter (about ⅓ of an inch or the size of a small pearl), the risk of cancer appears to be 0 to 2 percent. For polyps that measure 1 to 2 centimeters (up to ¾ of an inch or the size of a large grape), the cancer risk appears to be 10 to 20 percent. Polyps of more than 2 centimeters hold a cancer risk of 30 to 50 percent. Cancer also is more likely to develop in villous adenomas than in tubular adenomas or tubulovillous adenomas. However, some adenomas might never grow and become malignant.

Benign polyps might simultaneously coexist with cancer elsewhere in the colon and rectum. These are known as synchronous lesions. If a polyp is discovered during flexible fiberoptic sigmoidoscopy, which sees the lower third of the colon, it is good medical practice to then examine the entire colon with colonoscopy, a similar procedure that uses a longer instrument, to discover any simultaneously occurring polyps or cancers. In general, someone with a tendency to form colonic or rectal polyps is also at a higher risk of developing colon and rectal cancer.

Most patients who have polyps have no symptoms to warn of their presence. Thus polyps are likely to remain undiscovered and undiagnosed until the colon and rectum are inspected by colonoscopy, sigmoidoscopy, or barium enema X-ray. In rare cases, polyps might cause occult (hidden) amounts of blood to appear in the stool or might actually cause hemorrhage from the anus. Even more rarely, patients might complain of abdominal discomfort when a polyp stalk is subjected to peristaltic action (digested matter passing through) and "tugs" at the colon wall. If the polyp is very large, usually in the several-centimeter range, a blockage of the colon or rectum might occur and cause a person such distension or discomfort that it comes to the attention of the physician.

Three-quarters of adenomatous polyps and cancers are found in the left, or sigmoid colon. Left-sided adenomas are more likely to be detected by fiberoptic endoscopy, and naturally are more likely to come to a physician's attention. However, the frequency of many smaller adenomas in the right colon, which can be seen only with a colonoscopy, increases with age, especially after sixty.

Inside the Colon Wall   The lining of the colon undergoes constant regrowth of cells and renews itself completely every week. This process of cell growth—proliferation and differentiation—is highly regulated. Cells are produced, they mature, and they die at a regulated pace, so that the lining of the colon remains at the same thickness and maturity within a healthy mix of cell types.

However, when the cells disregard this process and begin to multiply and change character, the lining of the colon changes, and this can be observed endoscopically. Now the lining, or epithelium, has a characteristic look called dysplasia. This means that the epithelial cells are not behaving normally. This can be an early sign of malignancy and always raises a red flag to the gastroenterologist and pathologist. Polyps with severe dysplasia can become malignant in fewer than four years.

Another change that can be observed is hyperplasia, the excessive growth of a single layer of cells, which becomes several cell layers thick. Although the cells are not malignant, they are atypical and could change. Because these conditions indicate unusual cell activity, they must be treated with the same thoughtfulness as true colon cancers. Premalignant conditions can remain localized (contained within an area) until they develop into either noninvasive cancer or invasive cancer. Then there is the potential for spread into surrounding tissue or even the rest of the body. Hyperplastic polyps are not premalignant but cannot be diagnosed as hyperplastic until they are removed and biopsied.

Adenocarcinomas

Exactly how a polyp progresses to cancer still is not known, but most polyps seem to take from three to seven years to become malignant. The potential for the polyp to become cancerous depends on its size, type, and degree of atypia. This is why regular screenings are so important. These polyps should be found and removed before they become cancerous. Some polyps are small with low-grade cell growth and pose no immediate danger. Others are fast-growing and aggressive and can spread to other organs.

Morton, fifty-three, was reluctant to follow his wife's advice and get a surveillance colonoscopy. He had no symptoms and as far as he knew there was no colon cancer in his family. At his latest annual physical exam, there was no sign of disease from blood tests. As it turned out, Morton did have a small polyp, 1.5 centimeters, that was removed and found to be cancerous. Luckily, the cancer had not spread, and Morton was cured. Now he has become so convinced of the importance of surveillance that he urges all his friends to do it.

The chance of a polyp becoming cancerous increases 2½ to 4 times if the polyp is larger than 1 centimeter—⅓ of an inch—in diameter. The chance increases to 5 to 7 times if multiple polyps are present. The natural history of a polyp larger than 1 centimeter left untreated shows that the progression to cancer increases 2.5 percent at 5 years, 8 percent at 10 years, and 24 percent at 20 years. This progression also depends on the degree of dysplasia, or what the cells are doing. With severe dysplasia, the progression can be as few as 3.5 years, and with mild dysplasia, it might take more than 11 years.

Patients who have one adenoma are 30 to 50 percent more likely to have at least one more somewhere in the colon. Because multiple primary lesions (polyps) occur so often, a total colonoscopy is an essential part of the workup if a lesion is found during a more limited exam. If there are multiple lesions in the colon, they are generally synchronous lesions—those that occur at different times. These can be near one another or in different parts of the colon.

People with familial polyposis syndromes, ulcerative colitis, or a previous history of colon cancer are more likely to have synchronous polyps.

Patients with at least two synchronomous adenomas are also likely to have metachronous adenomas—that is, they are at increased risk to develop more polyps later. Part of the importance of finding and removing a polyp is that the doctor has identified a patient who will need surveillance for early detection of additional polyps and possibly colon cancer.

What to Know before an Endoscopic Biopsy

For purposes of a biopsy, part or all of a polyp can be removed or a piece of the colon lining can be removed. One of the benefits of colonoscopy is that the polyp can be removed when it is discovered in a low-risk procedure. The predunculated polyp has a stalk and is easily removed at the base with a wire snare through which an electric current is passed, permitting the polyp to be cauterized. The sessile polyp, on the other hand, has no stalk, and sometimes it cannot be completely removed either because it is not raised from the mucosa or because it is too small. When they are encountered, sessile polyps should be extensively biopsied or "shaved." The resulting fragments must be recovered and sent to the pathologist.

Only a small percentage of polyps show cancer, but all colonic polyps must be distinguished from carcinomas, and complete biopsies are critical. If a polyp is too large—bigger than 3 or 4 centimeters, or 1½ inches—only a piece of it might be removed. A 2-centimeter polyp that is flat cannot always be removed as easily as a pedunculated polyp that is attached to the colon wall by a stalk.

It is important to know what kind of polyp was removed and if it was completely or only partially removed. Partial biopsy could be misleading. If one piece of polyp is okay, there still could be cancer cells in the other part of the polyp. Ask your doctor about this.

Also, if a polyp with a stalk is removed and part of the stalk remains attached to the colon lining, another biopsy might be needed if cancer was found in the polyp. It is important to be sure no cancer has escaped into the remaining stalk. However, there are many "ifs" for patient and doctor to consider. Some medical literature claims removal of a polyp is enough. But some patients and doctors might ask about whether the stalk was cut straight. What if invasive cancer cells have passed through that stalk into the lining? This is why it is so important for patients to review pathology findings thoughtfully with their doctors, and to get a second opinion if necessary, possibly from a colorectal surgeon.

An extremely rare complication of removing a polyp is hemorrhage from the vessel that supplies blood to the body of the polyp. Another possible complication is perforation—formation of a hole—in the wall of the colon. The removal of large sessile polyps, as opposed to small to moderate-size pedunculated polyps, is more likely to predispose the patient to these complications.

Under the Microscope

When the pathologist studies the colonic tissue under the microscope, many things are revealed. The tumor size is measured. The edges of the polyp are checked to see if the tumor extends to those edges, or "margins." The most important job for the pathologist is to determine the depth of invasion, but a thorough analysis of the polyp or colonic tissue requires many studies.

The tumor cells are examined to determine if they are invasive, how fast they are growing, and how aggressive they are. If the cancer is invasive, further tests might be done. These pieces of information—the variables of colon cancer—are called prognostic indicators. They help guide both patient and doctors with decision-making about treatment. For example, approximately 20 percent of colon carcinomas are poorly differentiated or undifferentiated tumors. This means that the cells are aggressive and likely to invade other organs. Most carcinomas secrete a small or moderate amount of mucin, but about 10 to 20 percent of tumors are described as mucinous or colloid carcinomas because they produce large amounts of mucin. Mucinous carcinomas also are more aggressive. The grade of a cancer labels the overall pattern of the tumor cells and nuclei. It also tells how aggressive the cancer is. If it is Grade 1, then it is the least aggressive form. Grade 3 is the most aggressive and the most common.

Some of the things a patient should expect to see in a pathology report include depth of invasion, type and grade of carcinoma, and evidence of vascular invasion or invasion of the stalk or submucosa. A biopsy after abdominal surgery to remove the diseased piece of colon should also include the status of the margins on a resected piece of colon and the presence or absence of cancer cells in the lymph nodes.

The Polypectomy Procedure

Preparations for a polypectomy are the same as preparations for a colonoscopy, so you can refer back to chapter 3 and read the section on screening for diagnosis. Be sure you have a complete understanding of the procedure, so ask as many questions of your physicians as you need.

Before asking you to consent to the procedure, your doctor will caution you and tell you what to do about the risk of possible bleeding following the procedure. Bleeding can occur during the procedure, but the doctor can easily control this. Hemorrhage following polypectomy often requires hospitalization and might even require blood transfusion.

Expert polypectomy technique must be applied by the gastroenterologist, and the site will be recorded and might be marked with sterilized India ink so the surgeon can find it if you should need open abdominal surgery. A careful written assessment and description of the polyp and its location also must be supplied by the gastroenterologist. Because the colon is so flexible, the surgeon might not always find the polyp exactly where it shows up in the pictures taken by the endoscopic camera.

The polyp is encircled with a wire snare; then an electrocauterizing current passes through the endoscopic tube, and the polyp is removed. This might be all the treatment you need. However, it is critical to follow through with a biopsy and monitored surveillance with periodic colonoscopy to survey the entire colon for additional polyps. If you had one polyp, you are at higher risk to develop more.

After a thorough biopsy of the polyp is made by the pathologist, the information is communicated to your other physicians. Your gastroenterologist, pathologist, and surgeon must cooperate to assess the information about your colon cancer. Even with great care, it is possible for some polyps, especially sessile polyps without stalks and those removed piecemeal, to be inaccurately assessed for margin of resection and depth of invasion.

After a Polypectomy

After the uncomplicated discovery and removal of an adenomatous polyp of the colon or rectum, you will need to follow up with a colonoscopy, usually at two- to three-year intervals. And in the years when colonoscopy is not performed, your doctors might recommend that you have a complete blood count to watch for any change in tumor marker levels and that you are tested for hidden blood in the stool. If the polyp was particularly large or if multiple polyps were present, your doctor might modify this and recommend more frequent screening with colonoscopy.

The need for such surveillance cannot be overemphasized, because once you have had a cancerous polyp, you are at a three to four times greater risk of developing a second primary cancer of the colon. If another polyp develops and shows a cancer, it can be removed the same way, or a surgical colon resection can be done. If cancer is detected early, even the second time around, it usually can be cured with surgery.

Familial Polyposis Syndromes

Familial polyposis syndromes are hereditary conditions that include familial adenomatous polyposis (FAP), Gardner syndrome, Turcot syndrome, Peutz-Jeghers syndrome, Cowden disease, and familial juvenile polyposis.

The genetic condition known as familial polyposis syndrome (FAP) causes thousands of polyps to develop along the entire inside of the colon. It is caused by mutations in the adenomatous polyposis coli (APC) gene. Adenomatous polyps either sporadic or secondary to familial polyposis syndromes are the only premalignant type of polyp. Because there is no known way to prevent familial polyposis from developing, the only treatment is to remove the colon so polyps cannot develop. This prophylactic surgery is performed in adults as soon as the disease is diagnosed and in children when they reach their late teens. Each polyp is a step toward cancer. With so many polyps, sometimes thousands, a person's risk of developing colorectal cancer is almost 100 percent by age forty. It is usually unnecessary to operate before age twenty because most people with this syndrome do not develop the cancer until then. The treatment in young people is almost always accomplished easily without complications by using either the standard method or the J-pouch method.

People with the hereditary nonpolyposis colorectal cancer (HNPCC) syndrome (also known as Lynch syndrome) also are at high risk for colorectal cancer, although they do not develop polyps in the same number as in the FAP syndrome. Other cancers are common in people with HNPCC syndrome, including cancers of the uterus, ovary, stomach, small intestine, and breast. Four HNPCC genes have been discovered.

All members of a family do not have the same height or weight or facial features. And all members do not get the same diseases or susceptibility to them. Some will inherit genes that predispose to colorectal cancer; some will not. Memorial Sloan-Kettering Cancer Center in New York maintains a registry of patients and their families who have a strong medical history of either FAP or HNPCC. This is part of an international collaborative effort to identify and follow these individuals. It helps researchers as well as the families involved learn more about the disease.

Prophylactic Surgery for Familial Adenomatous Polyposis

The standard treatment for FAP is surgical removal of the entire colon and the joining of the small intestine directly to the rectum. Once the patient's digestive system has had a few months to adjust to the shortened intestine, normal bowel function resumes.

The J-pouch method was first used in the 1980s and still is a highly specialized procedure. The surgeon removes both the colon and the mucous membrane of the rectum without harming the rectal sphincter muscle. This muscle will be joined to the lower end of the small intestine, which will be transformed into a saclike reservoir or pouch to imitate the reservoir function of the rectum.

Surgeons seem to like the J-pouch for FAP and chronic ulcerative colitis patients, but it is less used in a colon cancer resectioning. For this, it is necessary to operate twice. During the first surgery, the colon is removed and a J-pouch created, even though it cannot be used right away. The small intestine is brought outside, onto the surface of the abdomen— an ileostomy—and for three months, stools will be eliminated through this stoma into a bag. Then the ileostomy will be removed, and the feces allowed to pass through the anus again.

In rare cases, where the patient has already developed cancer of the rectum before the detection of polyposis, the only possible treatment is a colostomy. About two months after this operation, all polyps in the rectum are removed by polypectomy during a sigmoidoscopy, which will be required from one to four times a year for the rest of the patient's life to immediately remove the new polyps that will continue to appear. Otherwise the patient is at risk for the development of rectal cancer.

The J-pouch method eliminates the risk of developing new polyps in the rectum, but it takes the patient six to twelve months to attain normal bowel movements. Once a year, the pouch will be examined with an endoscope.

When FAP is found and treated early, the patient lives a perfectly normal life with no urinary or sexual system disorders. Women who have had a J-pouch or standard surgery for FAP have just as much chance of getting pregnant and going through childbirth without complications as any other woman, although a cesarean birth is advisable after a J-pouch operation. In addition, all examinations, except for the X-ray study of the colon, can be carried out safely.

Colon Cancer

If colon polyps are found and removed early, through regular screening, colon cancer can be prevented. But until recent years, colon cancer was often fatal because nobody talked about it or would undergo screening. When our book *What to Do If You Get Colon Cancer* was published in 1996, it was the first one for the general public to take the fear and mystery from this disease and explain treatment options and prevention. This section includes some of that information, but if you or a family member has colon cancer, the earlier book will provide much more specific guidance.

Colon cancer evolves from a precancerous benign lesion or polyp that remains in the large intestine and grows. The goal of colon cancer prevention is to interrupt that process and to find and remove the polyp or tumor before it becomes cancerous. Or, if it is in the early stage of cancer, it can be cured before it has a chance to spread. The majority of colon cancers detected by screening programs are cured. Yet only half of all colon cancer cases are diagnosed at the curable stage. If we can only convince more people to get regular screenings, such as an annual digital exam, fecal occult blood test, complete blood count, periodic sigmoidoscopy, and in some people colonoscopy, we can knock colon cancer off the list of killers.

It has been estimated that half the population over fifty have colon polyps, and 95 percent of colon and rectal cancers originate with such polyps. We know this from autopsy studies, which also show that the number of polyps found varies widely among regions of the world. Several European countries have higher rates than the United States, but in most developing nations, the rate is considerably lower. In the United States, the incidence of colon cancer is greater in the North and in the East and lower in the South and in the West.

Colon cancer and rectal cancer are major health problems in the United States with more than 200,000 new cases diagnosed each year (135,000 are colorectal; 98,200 colon). They kill nearly 60,000 Americans every year. In adult men, these cancers are second only to lung cancer. In adult women, they are the third most prevalent cancers after breast cancer and lung cancer. The good news is that while the number of cases is increasing, the mortality rate is dropping, so more people are getting early detection and successful treatment.

When our hearts are not working, we feel a pain in the chest or shortness of breath. We know when something is wrong. But when something is wrong with the colon, we can be unaware of it for years. And even when we have symptoms, it is easy for a patient—or even a less than diligent health-care worker—to blame it on other conditions, such as diverticulosis, colitis, hemorrhoids, or irritable bowel syndrome.

Because vague abdominal discomfort is so common, the symptoms of colon cancer can often be confused with those of benign conditions, and patients sometimes fail to pursue thorough diagnostic screenings. It is far easier to diagnose a patient who has had a regular bowel movement at the same time every morning for forty years and now, for some reason, is having a different experience. Something tangible must have caused that change. But the patient who always has had bowel problems is going to be more difficult to diagnose. Even those previously treated for colonic ailments identified as benign are not protected from the development of colon cancer.

Colon cancer, rectal cancer, colorectal cancer—they are all the same disease. When we use the words *colon cancer*, we mean any cancer in the colon—from the cecum, at the beginning of the colon, to the rectum, the lowermost portion of the colon. (Because of the location of the rectum, treatment is sometimes different.)

It is important to understand the role of the colon in the mechanics of the digestive system. If you are going to need surgery for colon cancer, your entire digestive system will be shut down for several days, and understanding how that system works will better prepare you to cope with all the procedures involved in your treatment and follow-up care. Go back to chapter 1 for a detailed description of this.

In Situ or Invasive Cancer

Cancer is either in situ or invasive. In situ means "in place," contained within the polyp. The cancer has not broken through the colon wall into surrounding muscle and fat. Thus it is noninvasive.

Invasive, or infiltrating cancer, can break through or already has broken through the stalk of the polyp or through the colon wall into blood vessels, the lymph system, surrounding fatty tissue, or other organs. If the cancer is invasive, lymph nodes around the colon must also be examined to find out if the cancer has begun to spread elsewhere. Lymph fluids flow through the body like the bloodstream, and the bean-shaped lymph nodes are like filters, catching what comes through the system. As part of the immune system, they filter out and get rid of foreign or abnormal cells. It is here that colon cancer cells are likely to travel on their way to other organs.

Metastatic Cancer

Metastatic means the cancer has spread through the lymphatic system or the bloodstream to adjacent and/or distant tissues. Sites of local metastasis of colon cancer are usually lymph nodes. The liver and lungs are the most common distant sites for metastasis, followed by the adrenals, the ovaries in women, and then bone. Metastasis to the brain is rare.

Other Cancers That Rarely Occur in the Colon

Lymphomas can cause lymph nodes to enlarge and form a mass in the colon. Sometimes what appears to be an adenomatous polyp in the colon is not colon cancer at all, but cancer of the lymph system. The cancer can be primary—starting in the lymphatic tissue in the abdomen—or systemic—the colon mass is only one of the lymphoma tumors throughout the body. Colonic lymphomas account for less than 0.5 percent of all colon malignancies and are treated differently than colon cancers.

Sarcomas are rare malignancies that might arise from the colon lining. Kaposi's sarcoma has become more common with the emergence of AIDS and appears as a complication of that disease, involving about 75 percent of AIDS patients. The stomach and duodenum are more common sites for these sarcomas, but about a third of patients also get them in the colon.

There are other rare tumors that appear in the colon or rectum, including colloid carcinoma, signet ring cell carcinoma, adenosquamous carcinoma, and oat cell carcinoma.

Understanding the Risk Factors for Colon Cancer

Your medical history is extremely important to your doctor in diagnosis. Most doctors make a clear distinction between patients at risk for colon cancer because of age and those with diseases that predispose them to colorectal cancer. Additional risk factors include a personal history of colonic or rectal polyps, a family history of such polyps, a personal or family history of colon or rectal cancer, and certain other bowel and nonbowel conditions. The lifetime risk of an adult developing colon cancer is about 5 percent. From this baseline a number of risk factors can be identified.

Aging
The mere act of aging enhances the likelihood of getting colon cancer. By forty, the number of people getting this cancer each year begins to accelerate, doubling every decade until about eighty. For the majority—about 70 percent—of patients diagnosed with colon cancer, the only risk factor they have is their age. Age is the major determinant in frequency of colon cancer, with peak prevalence in men and women after sixty.

A Family Gene
In addition to the rare cases of hereditary colon cancer syndromes such as familial polyposis, there is more and more evidence that heredity plays a

major role in the development of colon and rectal cancer. The probability of colon cancer developing in a person who has a first-degree relative with this cancer is about 15 percent, as compared to a 5 percent risk in the general adult population. Studies have shown that patients with colonic polyps are two to five times more likely to have a first-degree relative with colon polyps. And those first-degree relatives are two to five times more likely to have colon cancer than the general population.

The National Polyp Study, lead by scientists at Memorial Sloan-Kettering Cancer Center in New York, concluded in 1996 that siblings and parents of patients with adenomatous polyps are at increased risk for colon cancer, particularly when the adenoma was diagnosed before age sixty, or in the case of siblings, when the parent has had colon cancer. Date from this study are expected to provide a basis for planning family-screening strategies.

Preexisting Bowel Conditions

Colon and rectal cancer can occur as a complication of inflammatory bowel disease, chronic ulcerative colitis, and to a lesser extent Crohn's disease. This is particularly so if the disease began early in life and has been present for more than fifteen years. Chronic ulcerative colitis (CUC) is the inflammation of part, or sometimes all, of the colon. About 5 percent of CUC patients will get colorectal cancer, and the longer they have this disease, the greater the risk.

Nonbowel Conditions

Genital and breast cancer in women have been proposed as high-risk factors for the development of colon cancer. Although there is no absolute proof of this connection yet, many physicians—especially oncologists—advise such patients to get regular screenings with sigmoidoscopy or colonoscopy.

Diet, Environment, and Race

Whether or not environment and diet are important risk factors for colon cancer remain to be proven, but they are taken into consideration because of the studies suggesting that geography and diet might factor into the incidence of colon cancer. For example, colon cancer risk is higher in African Americans than it is in native black African populations, suggesting again the impact of environmental factors. But is it genetic or environmental? Or both? Colon cancer incidence is low in Japanese men, but when these men move to Hawaii, the incidence of colon cancer increases dramatically. Is it the dietary switch from fish and rice to bacon and cheeseburgers?

There is no positive proof that diet—such as high-fat, low-fiber—alone is responsible for colon cancer. This is still being investigated. It is known that a low-fat, high-fiber diet is generally more healthful and prevents digestive problems as well. It appears that people who consume high amounts of fiber and who have large, bulky stools tend to have lower frequency of colon adenomas and cancers, possibly because waste matter moves through the colon faster. But it still is not known which types of fiber are involved and how much needs to be consumed.

Lack of Dietary Calcium

This also has been studied as a risk factor on the theory that calcium and vitamin D neutralize fatty acid created by a high-fat diet—much the way detergent cuts the grease in dishwater—and slow epithelial cell growth. Aspirin and related compounds also are under study, but the dynamics of the digestive system are too complicated for easy answers. For instance, the bacteria flora in the colon might oxidize bile acids that may have tumor-promoting activity. It will be years before studies produce hard facts in this area.

Alcohol Abuse

This increases the risk of all gastrointestinal cancers, including colon cancer. Alcoholism often results in lower intake of folate and other nutrients associated with certain oncogenes commonly implicated in colon cancer.

Symptoms of Colon Cancer

Because there are so many symptoms of colon diseases that overlap with colon cancer, it is easy to confuse the issue or to try to second-guess unless careful and methodical testing is done. More than a third of colon cancer patients studied had no symptoms. Symptoms usually do not occur until polyps become larger than one centimeter—about the size of your smallest fingernail—or until they crowd each other, as in the multiple polyps associated with familial polyposis syndromes. Symptoms such as constipation, diarrhea, flatulence, and painful bowel movements can also be symptoms of ulcerative colitis, irritable bowel syndrome, or diverticulosis.

A patient who has an annual physical during which anemia is discovered, for example, must identify the cause. It could range from blood loss from taking too many aspirins to menstruation. No problem is obvious. A doctor faced with a host of questions here and must rule out all other possibilities before making a diagnosis. First, the patient is questioned about possible reasons for loss of blood: Where there any changes in diet? In bowel habits? Could bleeding be caused by hemorrhoids, ulcerative colitis, or diverticulitis? Doctors must tease out suspicions from new-onset anemia and make their patients understand why further—and more invasive—tests are necessary.

Laura, a woman in her sixties, went to Egypt with three friends and took a cruise through the Nile region. All four women suffered from diarrhea, which they attributed to the food and water in their new environment. But while the other three women got better when they returned home, Laura did not. After listening to her account of what was wrong, the doctor had to ignore the travel story and look beyond that. Then through careful questioning, examination, and screening, it was found that Laura had colon cancer. It was only a coincidence that it developed at the time of the cruise.

June, a seventy-five-year-old woman, experienced vague abdominal discomfort and some constipation, but because she had been overindulging in food and wine during the holidays, she assumed her gastric discomfort was related to that. She took antacids, hoping to feel better. When she finally had a checkup, a malignant tumor was discovered high up in her colon, in the cecum.

When colon cancer is located in the right side of the colon, the cecum, the most common symptomatic complaints are abdominal pain that is usually dull and ill-defined, like June's was. Bleeding and weight loss also can occur. Colon cancer on the left side, or in the sigmoid area, manifests more often in changes in bowel habits, an increased use of laxatives, bleeding, gas pain, constipation, or narrowing of the stool.

Most colon cancer symptoms—despite a similarity to other conditions—fall into the following areas:

1. *Obstruction.* Colon cancers commonly grow, and the tumor becomes larger than the inner passageway—or lumen. The colonic lumen is widest in the cecum and ascending colon on the right side of the abdomen, and obstruction is much less likely to occur there. However, in the transverse colon, which crosses the abdomen near the navel, and in the descending and sigmoid colons, on the left side of the abdomen, the passageway is narrower, and thus obstruction is more likely to

occur. If the colonic lumen is completely blocked, pressure builds and causes pain and swelling of the abdomen. Nausea and vomiting might occur if the obstruction is extreme.

2. *Bleeding.* As tumors expand into the passageway, they are traumatized by the fecal stream, and this causes them to bleed. If the tumor is near the anus, the blood might be visible. But it is much more common for the blood to be hidden in stool. If such bleeding continues for months, it can cause iron deficiency anemia, evidence of which is sought therefore in making a diagnosis. But although bleeding is the most common symptom of colon cancer, only 20 percent of patients with rectal bleeding have colon cancer. Bleeding can mean any number of things, including hemorrhoids.

3. *Pain.* When invasive cells from the tumor eventually penetrate the wall of the colon and invade adjacent tissue, pain is felt, and other specific symptoms, depending on the organ invaded, appear. For example, if cancer cells penetrate into the bladder, urinary symptoms might appear. Sometimes physicians are drawn to the liver or bone because of a patient's pain and only later find a primary tumor in the colon, where it has produced hardy any symptoms at all.

4. *Wasting Syndrome.* Some tumors cause loss of appetite and decreased weight and strength. This can be all out of proportion to the size of the tumor, so there is much to investigate. The good news is that today, doctors have much better diagnostic tools than they did years ago. They can view the entire digestive system with sophisticated endoscopic equipment and easily take tissue samples for biopsy to more efficiently determine if cancer is present.

Diagnosis of Colon Cancer

Endoscopic screening procedures are not nearly as unpleasant as most people think. Even if you get regular annual physical checkups, it is not enough without the specific screenings for colon cancer. Physical examination, such as a digital rectal exam, by itself or palpating the abdomen, often does not detect signs of colon or rectal malignancy. Stool testing for occult blood and laboratory examinations such as blood count to detect anemia, iron levels, and liver blood tests provide some additional information. But the only sure way to find and identify polyps in the colon and rectum is with the barium enema X-ray; the flexible fiberoptic sigmoidoscopy, which examines the lower third of the colon and rectum; and the colonoscopy, which examines the entire colon.

A DNA stool test is under development. Expected to be widely available soon, this test examines the DNA found in stool to detect the presence of colorectal cancer or precancerous polyps. The test can be conducted at home and involves no advance preparation. It is painless and highly accurate—but not yet available. For complete explanations of these tests, refer to chapter 3.

Biopsy and Staging

The pathologist, a physician who specializes in the microscopic study (histology) of human tissue, is a very important part of the treatment team for colon cancer. There is much to be learned from the study of a polyp or tissue from the colon lining, and this information is critical to diagnosis and treatment. The pathologist might come to the endoscopic suite during a colonoscopy and polypectomy to discuss with the gastroenterologist the preparations for biopsy. These two physicians work together in interpreting their findings and staging the cancer.

If the pathologist discovers cancer in a polyp or in the cells of the colon or rectal mucosa, then the most important determination will be whether the cancer has penetrated the colon lining and wall. And if the cancer is invasive—meaning it has broken through the colon wall or has the potential to do so—then a surgical biopsy of lymph nodes and a section of the colon might be necessary because it gives the doctors a chance to get the most information microscopically about what is going on. And they also can look at the cancer and surrounding tissue with their own eyes. This is called gross examination.

The Surgical Biopsy

Once it has been determined that cancer has invaded the colon wall, more pathological examinations will be done after surgery.

Colon resection   The section of the colon that is removed during surgery is sent to a lab, where it is measured and tested for a number of indicators. As a matter of routine, the pathologist will look to see if the tumor involved the "edges" of what the surgeon removed. If so, that generally means cancer has spread. Distal and proximal margins are anatomical locations on the piece of colon resected. Distal is toward the rectum, and proximal is toward the cecum. Generally, the only time the proximal and distal margins are both positive for cancer is when the disease is lying low in the colon, near the rectum and sphincter muscle. In that tightly congested area, it is not possible to remove a large enough section of colon to allow for clean margins. Then removal of the rectum and a colostomy usually is necessary.

Lymph nodes   Some lymph nodes around the colon section also will be removed for study. These lymph nodes usually are found in the mesenteric layer of fat around the colon and are early indicators of whether cancer has spread from the colon. These nodes are a critical prognostic factor of a patient's diagnosis. Are they negative or positive for cancer? The number of lymph nodes analyzed depends on the size of the piece of colon removed.

It is possible to have a large colon cancer tumor and no affected lymph nodes. Each case must be treated individually. If the cancer has spread to the lymph nodes, it means there is an increased risk for systemic recurrence of colon cancer. Any lymph node showing cancer is evaluated to see if the cancer is contained inside the node or has broken through the shell of the node. A pathologist might examine, on average, about ten lymph nodes. For some reason, there are usually more lymph nodes around the right colon, the cecum, and fewer on the left side, around the sigmoid colon. Lymph node status, along with tumor size, are two of the most important prognostic indicators, crucial to treatment planning. With even one lymph node showing cancer, a patient should talk with a medical oncologist about the risk of systemic and local recurrence of colon cancer and whether chemotherapy is needed.

Interpreting Your Pathology Reports

Surprisingly, few patients ask to see their pathology reports. These written reports are sent by the pathologist to the gastroenterologist or surgeon, who tells the patient what it says and puts it in his or her file. You can ask for your own copy of the report so you can ask questions about what it contains. This report gives you information that you need to understand treatment, and you should become familiar with it. For example, the study of the cells in your tumor can affect choices or dosages of medications to use in chemotherapy. Ask your gastroenterologist, surgeon, or oncologist to tell you what everything means in these reports and how the doctors interpret the report. Take it with you if you talk with other doctors for additional opinions.

The first biopsy report will tell you about your polyp or tumor, and subsequent operative reports will evaluate your lymph nodes and a colon section. It should take no more than seven days from the time of biopsy until receipt of the report. Doctors often hear a preliminary report from the pathologist by phone, so you might have some information sooner.

How Colon Cancer Is Staged

Once your biopsies—endoscopic and surgical—have been completed, your cancer can be staged. This is a rather elaborate classification system based on the sum of many variables. Everything your doctors have learned about your colon cancer, from its physical appearance through all the tests—are classified and subclassified: size, type, location of tumor, depth of invasion, cell activity. Stage is generally the most important prognostic indicator.

Most cancers are categorized in Stages 1 through 4, but colon cancer staging is generally categorized in a system known as Dukes, which is more specific. In general, Stages 1 through 4 relate to Duke's A to D.

Duke's Classification

The stage of the colon cancer and your general health help determine your treatment options. A system called Modified Duke's Classification is the one most widely used to stage colon cancer:

- *Duke's Stage A* is cancer in situ or high-grade dysplasia and means cancer is limited to the mucous membrane that lines the colon. Five-year survival rate after treatment is 90 percent.

- *Duke's Stage B1* means cancer has penetrated into but not through the muscularis propria, a deeper layer of the colon wall. Five-year survival rate after treatment is 80 percent.

- *Duke's Stage B2* means cancer has penetrated through the muscularis propria or the serosa, the outer lining of the colon wall. Five-year survival rate is 70 percent.

- *Duke's Stage B3* is local extension of the primary tumor to another organ including the abdominal wall.

- *Duke's Stage C1* is the same as B1 plus lymph node metastasis. Five-year survival rate after treatment is 50 percent.

- *Duke's Stage C2* is the same as B2 plus lymph node involvement. Five-year survival rate is 50 percent.

- *Duke's Stage D* means there is distant metastasis. Survival rate after treatment is generally less than five years.

The TNM System

Another system physicians use to provide uniform pathologic categories is the TNM System—tumor, nodes, metastasis:

Tumor

- T is carcinoma in situ.
- T1 indicates submucosal invasion (Duke's Stage A).
- T2 indicates invasion of the muscularis propria (Duke's Stage B1).
- T3 indicates invasion through the muscularis propria into the subserosa or perirectal tissues (Duke's Stage B2).
- T4 indicates invasion into adjacent organs or tissues (Duke's Stage B3).

Nodes

- N0 means no involved lymph nodes.
- N1 means one to three regional nodes are involved (Duke's Stage C1).
- N2 means more than three regional lymph nodes are involved (Duke's Stage C2).
- N3 means a metastasis along the course of a major blood vessel.

Metastasis

- M0 means no distant metastasis.
- M1 means metastasis is present.

The grade of the cancer also is a significant influence in prognosis. For example, patients whose cancers are Grades 1 and 2 have better five-year survival rates than those with Grade 3.

The location of the tumor is an independent factor. Among patients with the same-stage disease, rectal carcinomas might be more difficult to cure than carcinomas in the colon. And in the colon itself, transverse and descending colon carcinomas seem to result in poorer outcomes than those in the ascending or sigmoid colon.

Ask your physician how he or she arrived at your particular staging. Although there are more precise and standard guidelines, there are always situations that might fall between two categories, so it is sometimes a judgment call by the doctor.

Treating Colon Cancer: Before You Begin

Colon cancer treatment is fairly straightforward and offers fewer options than treatments for breast or prostate cancer. Nevertheless, you have to make some decisions now. Generally, if your cancer is invasive and has broken through the colon wall, a section of the colon must be removed. This means major surgery. The second biopsy after surgery will help decide if chemotherapy is necessary.

Both treatment and prognosis of colon and rectal cancer depend on the depth of invasion of the cancer, the involvement of adjacent lymph nodes, and the presence or absence of distant metastases. Your treatment might involve local excision, polypectomy (a minor surgical procedure to remove the polyp), or open abdominal surgery to remove all or part of your colon. It also might include chemotherapy and, if you have rectal cancer, radiation as well.

Suppose you are told that you need open abdominal colorectal surgery. It is quite likely that your gastroenterologist will recommend the best treatment and surgeon if you need one. But do not be rushed. This procedure requires disruption of your lifestyle, at least a week's recovery in the hospital, and several more weeks of recuperation at home. Now is the time to get all the information and support you need, as well as a second or third opinion. See chapter 2 for additional information about getting more opinions.

Surgical Treatment: Local Excision, Polypectomy

Both treatment and prognosis of colon and rectal cancer depend on the depth of invasion of the cancer, the involvement of adjacent lymph nodes, and the presence or absence of distant metastases. In general, surgical treatment cuts away the tumor; then a course of adjuvant chemotherapy follows to catch any possible lingering cancer cells or to prevent their return. In cases of rectal cancer, radiation often is added after surgery to rid the area of the threat of metastasis.

There are slight variations on these treatments that will be explained as we go along. But it is most important to be sure you fully understand the rationale behind the treatment your doctors recommend. Within certain boundaries, colon cancer treatment should be individualized after taking into account a patient's extent of disease, lifestyle, and needs, not to mention age, occupation, and personal philosophy. For example, a police officer who wears a gun in a holster or a bus driver who wears a seat belt would do well to avoid a colostomy if possible because the holster or belt would press against the colostomy appliance. However, if it cannot be avoided, a surgeon can measure that officer or bus driver in uniform and while going through the motions of their jobs. Often, the surgery can be planned so as to avoid any undue stress on the appliance.

Surgical treatment—local excision and polypectomy or colon resection—usually is recommended for all Stage A, B, and C prognoses, unless the patient is at an extremely high risk for surgery; that is, the patient has other medical conditions, such as heart disease, drug addiction, or obesity that could add to the risk of anesthesia or the trauma of open surgery.

Following surgery, chemotherapy will be offered to virtually all patients with Duke's Stage C cancer and sometimes for Duke's Stage B cancer, but this is an area of controversy. Some physicians believe surgery is sufficient for these stages because the chance of the cancer having spread elsewhere is so low that putting the patient through the expense and possible discomfort of chemotherapy treatment are not practical.

Colorectal surgeons usually do not recommend surgery for Duke's Stage D cancer unless resection is required to control bleeding, relieve pain, protect adjacent organs, or prevent bowel obstruction. At this advanced stage, surgery also might be required to remove parts of other organs, such as the liver or ovaries, where the cancer might have spread. Chemotherapy or radiation treatments in patients with inoperable Duke's Stage D cancer have been marginally effective. But radiation therapy might be useful in relieving pain when the colon cancer has spread to the bones. Clinical trials of chemotherapy or biological therapy also are an option for patients at this stage.

Although it is not a general practice, some doctors try to shift the Duke's Stage by using preoperative radiation, sometimes in conjunction with chemotherapy, to shrink the tumor and thus improve surgical results with a lesser stage of cancer. Sometimes this is successful. It is not common to give preoperative radiation to change a classification, but it has been done, so it is mentioned here. The radiation treatment carries with it other potential problems. If your doctor suggests preoperative radiotherapy, ask many questions about the goal of treatment and get at least one more opinion.

Radiation treatment is primarily used for rectal cancer, which can present more complications because of its location. The rectum is surrounded by fat and by a network of nerves and blood vessels at the base of the spine that control sexual and voiding functions, among a host of others. If cancer is low in the rectum, a local excision can be done through the anus. Otherwise, rectal cancer requires an abdominal-perianal resection with the creation of a colostomy. This might be done with or without preoperative chemotherapy and/or radiation.

Treatment for Early Colon Cancer

Most early colon cancers—Duke's Stage A and B—can be cured by simply removing the cancer. This is done during a colonoscopy, for a colon cancer in a polyp, or with surgery.

If the cancer involves only the tip or mucosa of the polyp, the cancer, in essence, has been cured by the polypectomy and no further surgery is indicated. This situation is known as carcinoma in situ. A surveillance colonoscopy should be performed in six to twelve months.

If, in the opinion of the pathologist, the cancer is moderately or well differentiated, if it extends below the mucosa of the polyp but does not involve the blood vessels or lymphatics of the polyp stalk, the cancer probably has been cured by removal of the polyp. Open abdominal surgery with resection of the involved section of the colon is not indicated because the surgical risk is generally regarded as being higher than the risk of finding any residual cancer in the colon. Follow-up surveillance colonoscopy would be scheduled at six to twelve months after removal of the polyp.

If cancer is found to involve the resected margin of the stalk of the polyp, then cancer remains in the colon wall despite removal of the polyp, and surgical resection of the involved area of the colon is appropriate if the patient can undergo surgery. A repeat colonoscopy is performed three to six months later.

If the cancer has involved the blood vessels or lymphatics of the polyp, there is a risk that residual cancer cells might be present in or might have spread to the wall of the colon. Many physicians would recommend a segmental surgical resection of the colon if the patient is a good operative risk. If residual cancer is found in the colon wall at the time of surgical resection, a repeat colonoscopy for surveillance might be done in three to six months. If no residual cancer is found in the surgically resected colon wall, a colonoscopy would be done in six to twelve months.

When a Polypectomy Is all You Need

If cancer has not reached the edges of the polyp, it is not likely to threaten other organs. Research has shown that even when cancer is in the tip of the polyp, the likelihood that it has spread elsewhere is so minimal that a polypectomy is generally sufficient for cure.

However—and this is a big however—some physicians still prefer to remove the section of the colon that contained the polyp because they are uneasy about the possibility that there could be a micrometastasis in the colon wall or stalk of the polyp that would be discovered years later. Many patients, too, would rather have it out and be sure, even though colon resection means open abdominal surgery requiring an extended hospital stay and weeks of recuperation.

If you and your doctor decide that a polypectomy is sufficient, even with the presence of invasive cancer cells, you both need to assume some of the responsibility for possible undertreatment with this decision. You also must take into consideration your own ability to maintain surveillance. Are you sure you will be diligent about getting the necessary and frequent colonoscopies and fecal occult blood tests, and possibly other tests, to monitor your colon for possible return of cancer? Consider these questions seriously.

In general, a polypectomy is sufficient treatment for a cancerous polyp with invasive cells if:

- The polyp was not excised in a piecemeal fashion.
- Blood vessels and lymphatics do not appear to be involved.
- The colon wall is not invaded.
- No cancer shows at the margins of the resection (site of the removed polyp).

If cancer cells have invaded the polyp stalk or the lining of the colon wall or if there is evidence of blood vessels and lymphatic involvement, a colectomy (colon resection) would be a wise choice of treatment.

Local Excision for Rectal Cancer

Because there is so much fatty tissue between the rectum and the nearby organs, including the network of sacral nerves that control sexual function and bladder control, it is often assumed that microscopic tumor cells could be lurking in this congested area, ready to invade other parts of the body. Although sophisticated colorectal surgery can spare the sphincter muscles and sometimes the vital sacral nerves as well, the general surgical rule is to cut away as wide a margin as possible—just to be safe.

If you have a small rectal carcinoma of fewer than 3 centimeters in diameter (1¼ inches), if your biopsy reveals that the cells are not fast-growing, and if the lesion is mobile when it is examined, you might have the option of a local excision without open abdominal surgery and lymphadenectomy.

This surgery can be performed transanally or with a posterior proctotomy. In many cases, deep resection and/or fulguration (burning away the tumor in multiple, staged attacks, with electrical cauterization) of the base of the polyp can be performed under general or spinal anesthesia, through the anus, with the surgeon using a variety of instruments designed to shave the tumor and its roots.

Local excision is often substituted for open abdominal surgical resection of the involved section of colon. Many factors will help decide if this approach is appropriate for you. A second opinion also would be appropriate for this situation.

Radiation therapy is almost always a follow-up to this surgery to eliminate any possible lingering cancer cells in the pelvic area. When radiation is expected to follow rectal surgery, the surgeon will mark the area to be irradiated with large metal clips. This provides a guide for the radiation therapist in locating the tumor bed.

Surgical Treatment: Partial and Total Colectomy, Colostomy

When the diseased portion of the colon is cut away and the two healthy portions are reconnected, it is called a surgical resection. It is also called resectional surgery, colectomy, or hemicolectomy. Surgical techniques for rectal cancer are different, and they will be discussed later.

It is currently possible to resect the colon without fully opening the abdomen by using laparoscopic techniques. This involves inserting a tube through the abdominal wall, and with the aid of cameras and video screens performing surgery inside the abdomen by manipulating tools at the end of the tube. However, this type of surgery is not yet widespread for curing colon cancer. For one thing, the surgeon cannot see and feel the adjoining abdominal organs, especially the liver, and this is an important step in evaluating the disease and its treatment. In addition, the technique for this surgery requires formidable skills that few surgeons and medical centers currently have. So far, laparoscopic surgery has been primarily used to perform palliative therapy to reduce pain in patients with advanced colon cancer. But there are important clinical trials in progress.

Minimally invasive surgery involves insufflating the abdomen with carbon dioxide gas, which pushes the abdominal wall away from the intestine and allows the surgeon to work. Thin instruments and a magnifying video camera are placed into the abdomen and used for dissection. Instruments are placed in the abdomen through small incisions called ports. With the aid of video monitors, the surgeon and assistants can perform the operation.

With colon cancer, it is critical to remove the complete tumor as well as a margin of cancer-free space around it, and the draining lymph nodes. Many clinical trials have compared the size of the resection margin and the number of nodes removed after open or laparoscopic colectomy for cancer. No difference is seen, indicating that laparoscopic colectomy for cancer is feasible from a technical point of view. The concern was recurrence of cancer at the port site. A study of twenty-six hundred cases showed that port site recurrence was about 1 percent, which is similar to that for open surgery.

Laparoscopic surgery means quicker recovery time. The disadvantage is increased operative time—most are thirty to seventy-five minutes longer than for open surgery. The experience of the surgeon also is critical, and it takes time to learn how to do this. Studies show that the operative time decreases significantly if the surgeon has done a significant number of these procedures.

While laparoscopic surgery meant less recovery time, the outcome on the patient was no different than with open surgery.

About Open Abdominal Surgery

Traditional colorectal surgery is open abdominal surgery under general anesthesia. It includes not only resecting the colon, but also removing lymph nodes for analysis and investigating nearby organs, such as the liver, for signs of cancer. The length of colon removed depends on the size of the cancer and its location. Your surgeon will want to leave a wide margin on either side of the tumor, usually 4 centimeters, or $1\frac{1}{2}$ inches. Sewing the two healthy parts of the colon together is called anastomosis.

Removing the entire colon would be a colectomy, and removing the colon and rectum would be a proctocolectomy, resulting in an ileostomy. There are many labels for colon surgery, although they are all the same surgery. If your tumor is in the sigmoid colon (the descending colon), you will be treated with a left hemicolectomy, the most common type of colon cancer surgery.

Sleeve resection is the simplest resection. It is done in cases of a very small tumor, or with a frail person who will not tolerate open surgery well. The cancerous section is cut away, the healthy sections joined, and that is all. No lymph nodes are removed, nor are other organs investigated.

Getting Ready for Surgery

Within two weeks of surgery you might be scheduled for preoperative tests such as a chest X-ray, an EKG, and blood tests to check your general health to be sure you are able to tolerate surgery and general anesthesia. You will want to interview the anesthesiologist and find out what kinds of drugs will be used. Likewise, the anesthesiologist will want to know what if any medications you have been taking.

If you have current medical conditions, these need to be brought to the attention of all the physicians involved in your care and treatment. Some medical conditions present risk factors for surgery. Obesity and heavy smoking or drinking could preclude anesthesia.

Shutting Down the Digestive System

To assure successful surgery, it is important that your intestines be empty and clean. This is called "mechanical bowel prep" for elective surgery, as opposed to emergency surgery, and begins two days before surgery. In the past, a patient would come into the hospital the night before for this preparation, but now you do it at home and come in the morning of your surgery, ready to go to the operating room.

Your doctor will give you detailed instructions, but the procedure is something like this: Two days before surgery, you will stop eating solid food and begin a diet of clear liquids only. You might be required to drink citrate of magnesia or the lavage used for colonoscopy to clear out any remaining waste material. This substance turns fecal matter to liquid and flushes it from your body. You also might be asked to give yourself a self-administered enema the morning of surgery to remove any residual fecal matter.

The night before surgery, you might be required to take antibiotics to kill bacteria remaining in the colon. Another dose of antibiotics, this intravenously, might be given to you immediately before and right after surgery.

The Surgery

The nurses and anesthesiologist get you ready, paint your abdomen with antiseptic, and cover up the rest of your body with sterile drapes. During this time, the anesthesia will begin to relax you. Colon resection surgery and lymphadenectomy take about two hours. Formation of a colostomy might take slightly longer.

Incisions are generally drawn down the center of your abdomen, often from just above the navel to the pubis. Sometimes they begin higher up, closer to the sternum if the cancer is high in the colon. A transverse incision on the right or left side of your abdomen sometimes is used for right- or left-sided lesions. The layers of muscle, fat, and skin of your abdomen are separated and clamped to expose the organs inside.

Because the colon stretches and is free-floating, the cancer is not always found exactly where it showed up on the colonoscopy, so the surgeon must explore. What the colonoscopy shows is merely a guide. Gross examination—what the surgeon can see and feel—is very important in this kind of surgery. Once the incision is made, clamps are placed above and below the diseased portion of the colon, and the cancerous portion of the colon is cut out.

Variations on the surgery depend on your particular case and your surgeon.

The surgeon will look at the other parts of the intestines, the liver, and the pelvis. The full length of the large bowel will be examined. It should be palpated along every inch. In women, the ovaries also will be examined. All adjoining organs can be explored so the surgeon will know that if extensive disease if found, the nature of the surgery might change—it might call for a less radical resection than would be provided for a cure, and chemotherapy might be added later.

When the colon section is removed, the surgeon also will cut out a wedge of the mesentery, the film of tissue that contains blood vessels and lymph nodes that drain the colon. It is attached to the back of the abdomen wall and supports the intestines. Because the lymph nodes drain the colon, cancer cells would go to these nodes. Not only is the lymphadenectomy critical for staging, it also is therapeutic. If any lymph nodes do contain cancer, their removal has eliminated additional cancer from your body from that source.

Nearby organs. If nearby organs show cancer, they also may be removed. For example, 2 to 8 percent of women with colon cancer will eventually show metastasis to the ovaries. For this reason the ovaries sometimes are removed to prevent cancer there. This is routinely considered for post- or perimenopausal women.

Reconnecting the Colon

Because the colon stretches like a rubber band, it can be shortened and reconnected without too much impact on your digestive system. If anything, a shortened colon reduces constipation. Your colon will eventually adapt to the new, shorter length.

The inner and outer layers of your colon are stitched or stapled together. Surgeons have their own preferences for the method used. The standard method is stitching the inner layer with a watertight seal of catgut, which eventually dissolves, and the outer layer with silk thread, which is permanent. Layers of your abdominal muscle, fat, and skin might be sewn together with stitches or stapled. These details depend on the location of your resection and your surgeon's preference.

Surgical Treatment: Rectal and Recurring Cancer

About 20 to 25 percent of cancers of the large intestine are rectal cancers, and these are most common in people between ages fifty and seventy. Many patients with rectal cancer delay coming for treatment because they think they have hemorrhoids. Sometimes they do—but that does not mean they do not also have a carcinoma. Hemorrhoids are varicose veins that protrude from the anal lining and are aggravated by constipation and straining to pass stool.

One seventy-year-old man, who delayed visiting a gastroenterologist until he noticed large amounts of blood in his stool, insisted to the doctor that his hemorrhoids were bleeding. A sigmoidoscopy and biopsy revealed that he had a large cancerous tumor in his rectum. When surgery and adjuvant chemotherapy were prescribed, the man insisted that he just wanted the hemorrhoids removed.

The patient delayed treatment every step of the way because of his insistence that he did not have cancer and that he would not be able to "wear the bag," meaning the appliance needed with a colostomy. After many months of procrastination, and after losing weight and showing many other signs of cancer, he finally consented to surgery but still resisted the recommended follow-up chemotherapy. There is a variety of techniques that allow removal of the tumor while preserving the sphincter muscles, thus avoiding colostomy. The rectum is about five inches long and surrounded by fat, which is a particularly fertile breeding ground for cancer cells. Any invasion greater than Duke's Stage A requires a wide excision, usually combined with abdominal resection and colostomy. Usually this is not required for similar cancers higher in the colon.

Anterior Resection

Cancer of the upper rectum is easier to control and usually is treated with an anterior resection. This can be appropriate if the growth is more than 2½ inches from the anus. This procedure removes the tumor and some cancer-free bowel on either side. Then the remaining rectum is joined to the colon with a surgical stapling system. A staple gun is inserted into the rectum through the anus, where it delivers a ring of tiny metal staples that hold the edges of the rectum and the colon firmly together.

In general, a rectal tumor can be treated with an anterior resection, without a colostomy, if the lower edge is more than 8 centimeters (about

3 inches) from the anal verge in a woman or more than 9 to 10 centimeters (4 inches) from the anal verge in a man. When cancer is in the lower part of the rectum, the entire rectum and the anus must be removed and a colostomy done.

There also are a host of potential complications because of the location of the rectum. Nerves needed for sexual potency and continence are generally destroyed during surgical treatment for rectal cancer. To compound this, blood vessels that men need for penile erection are often destroyed in radiation treatment that commonly follows rectal surgery. Sometimes the coccyx at the base of the spine is removed to expose the rectum and facilitate resectioning.

A patient with a small rectal cancer tumor, even in the distal 6 centimeters, might refuse a proctectomy and colostomy because of the possible complications and changes in lifestyle that come with this operation. Or the patient might not be a suitable operative candidate. In this case, a local transanal excision of the tumor might be considered. This might be a less than optimal treatment, leaving the patient with a risk of recurrence.

Colostomy

This procedure is performed when removal of the tumor requires removal of the rectum. A colostomy is a new opening through which waste matter can pass. Only about 15 percent of colon cancer patients, or one in seven rectal cancer patients, receive a colostomy.

When the colon and rectum are removed, the small intestine—the ileum—is passed through an opening called a stoma in the abdomen wall. The result is a total colectomy or total proctocolectomy, which results in an ileostomy. This new opening in the abdomen wall becomes the stoma. Waste is eliminated through this stoma into a sleeve that can be emptied directly into the toilet or into a pouch fastened to your body. Vast improvements have been made in colostomy appliances, and it is not as difficult to live with as it was when the bags were bulky and made of rubber, which did not conceal odors very well.

Sometimes a temporary colostomy is needed to give the lower colon and rectum time to heal after surgery. A second operation is performed later, and the healthy sections of the colon are joined and the stoma removed. Then bowel function returns to normal.

What to Expect after a Colostomy

In the past the hospital stay after a colostomy was about three weeks, or until doctors were certain the patient could manage at home. Now the emphasis is on home care and patient responsibility. This means arranging for a home care nurse who comes daily for at least one week to check your vital signs, to see how your wound is healing, and to continue teaching you how to manage your colostomy appliances and procedures. Gradually the visits are cut back as the patient and family assume the responsibility.

In most large hospitals, a specially trained enterostomal therapy nurse will work with you after a colostomy and help you learn how to cope with the special appliances.

You will need to get used to having a stoma, an opening in your abdomen. The stoma is made of membrane, which looks much like the inside of your mouth, and can secrete mucus. It has blood vessels, so it can bleed if it is irritated. No matter how well prepared, the initial sight of the stoma is a shock to most patients, almost like a slap in the face. But with help from nursing specialists and support groups, you and your family can learn to adapt. Some hospitals arrange for an ostomy representative to visit you in the hospital before as well as following your surgery.

If you had a total colostomy, your feces will now pass directly from your small intestine through the stoma and into the colostomy pouch. Because there is no longer a colon to remove water from waste matter and make it solid, you will have liquid feces.

If any problem becomes severe or causes pain, be sure to report it to your nurse or doctor.

Side Effects of Rectal Surgery

Radical colorectal surgery to the rectum usually has side effects that cause lasting changes in your lifestyle. All of these side effects must be explained to you by your surgeon before you consent to the operation. The most serious side effects result when some of the sacral nerves are cut away. These nerves, centered at the base of the spine, nervate the thighs, buttocks, and muscles and skin of the legs and feet, as well as of the anal and genital areas. These nerves cannot be restored after surgery, so this is one reason why it is so important to understand exactly what your surgery means.

When the nerves are severed, it can cause sexual dysfunction in men. Less common, but also possible in men, it can cause urinary retention—that is, the nerves that make possible the reflex that allows the release of urine do not work.

Radiation treatment for this area of the body also can produce problems. Radiation is almost certain to destroy the blood vessels necessary for penile erection. Chemotherapy can limit the ability of the muscles in the genital area to function.

Sexual function can be restored in a variety of ways. Be sure you know all you can about these side effects so you can understand how you can treat these problems after your surgery.

Surgical Options for Metastatic and Recurring Colon Cancer

When colon cancer is advanced, the more common treatment would be chemotherapy to help reduce pain and improve the quality of life for the patient. Surgical resection of the colon would not cure the cancer, but it might be considered necessary to prevent further obstruction of the colon, to repair damage such as perforation, or to stop bleeding.

However, if the colon cancer has spread to the liver, there are surgical options for further treatment. If a single hepatic metastasis or group of lesions in a single lobe of the liver is discovered and there is no other evidence of metastasis, then surgical resection of the liver is considered the best option and might provide a long-term, disease-free, clinical course. Left untreated, a malignant lesion of the liver would soon be fatal.

Colon cancer usually spreads first to the lymph nodes and then to the liver through the blood vessels. The liver is the most common site of metastasis. It also is the first site of distant spread in about one-third of patients with recurrences and is involved in more than two-thirds of fatalities. Colon cancer rarely spreads to the lungs or lymph nodes around the clavicle or to less common areas such as bone or the brain without first involving the liver. The most notable exception to this generalization is in patients with a primary tumor in the lower part of the rectum. Tumor cells from lesions in that area can spread through the blood vessels around the spine and vertebrae and travel up to the lungs and supraclavicular lymph nodes at the juncture of the neck and shoulders.

This surgery is considered appropriate for patients whose primary tumor is controlled or controllable, who have fewer than five metastases in the liver, and who show no other sign of colon cancer. About 5 percent of patients who had colon surgery are suitable for this procedure, and they are generally younger, otherwise healthy people.

More and more, patients with isolated metastatic cancer of the liver can be identified early by the monitoring of their carcinoembryonic antigen tumor marker levels—CEA assay—through blood tests. Tumors do recur in about one-third of these patients.

Radiation Treatment for Rectal Cancer

Like surgery, radiation therapy is a local treatment. It treats only the area it directly touches. It is rarely used for colon cancer because radiation into the abdomen has not proven successful and can be toxic when combined with chemotherapy. However, radiation therapy plays an important role in the treatment of patients with Duke's Stage B and Stage C rectal tumors, and it is quite effective in curing the cancer or preventing recurrence.

There are several ways of using radiation to treat rectal cancer. It can be used before surgery to shrink the tumor, or it can be used after surgery to kill any lingering cancer cells. Researchers are studying the benefits of using it both before and after surgery—the sandwich technique—and even during surgery.

For most patients, the best time for radiation appears to be after surgery. Most radiation begins four to six weeks after surgery and is given daily on weekdays for five to seven weeks. The radiation is sent into the rectum through the pelvic area for only a few seconds, but after a week or two the pelvic area may swell and the skin become pink or deep red. The intensity varies with skin type. The boost is the final phase of treatment and is given during the last two weeks. The boost directs a dose of radiation directly into the tumor bed. This can be done externally, using the radiation machine, or internally, by implanting radioactive particles into the body.

Radiation can make you tired and listless, so get plenty of rest, but try to maintain as normal a life as possible. Most people continue to work and schedule treatments for early mornings or late afternoons.

When radiation therapy is completed, expect to have a routine checkup within two months. This will include a physical examination of the rectum to check the aftereffects of treatment and possibly a transrectal sonogram.

You also should see your surgeon at six-month intervals. You might alternate with your medical oncologist if you are taking cytotoxic chemotherapy. This close follow-up procedure continues for five years while the potential for recurrence is highest.

Radiation Combined with Chemotherapy

In treating rectal cancer, radiation might be used in combination with chemotherapy or used before or after chemotherapy. One study showed that compared with the same dose of radiation used alone, this combined regimen of radiation and chemotherapy reduced the recurrence rate by 33 percent and the death rate by 29 percent.

Side Effects of Radiation Therapy

The side effects of radiation therapy have a lasting impact on your lifestyle, so it is important that you understand what they actually involve, and how you can correct these side effects. Because of the location of vital blood vessels at the base of the spine, it is impossible to prevent damage during radiation treatment. Even if the nerves in this area were spared by conservative surgery, the effects of radiation to those blood vessels cannot be prevented.

Chronic damage to the small bowel or bladder is uncommon, but men might become impotent because radiation damages the blood vessels that carry blood to the penis for an erection. Similarly, vessels that carry blood to the genital area in women during sexual arousal might not function as well and result in vaginal dryness.

However, this does not mean you will no longer have a sex life. It simply means that men will have to adapt to new ways of achieving an erection, and women may need to use a lubricant during intercourse. It is very important to discuss this openly with your doctor and your partner to learn how to deal with it.

Other side effects of radiation to the rectum include gastrointestinal symptoms such as nausea and diarrhea; hair loss in the pelvic area, which could be permanent; skin irritation; fatigue; and the slight risk of getting cancer again from the radiation.

When You Need Chemotherapy

Colon cancer cells are resistant to chemotherapy and they respond only to variations on two drug regimens that have been in use since 1989, when a particular combination of drugs dramatically increased survival rates. A new class of drugs has been introduced in the twenty-first century, and these drugs sometimes are combined with traditional ones. The course of chemotherapy for colon cancer most commonly takes a year, but each case is unique. Sometimes six months might be enough; sometimes it takes longer. The good news is that the side effects are generally not as intense as they can be with drugs used for other cancers.

Chemotherapy is standard treatment for Duke's Stage C colon cancer and sometimes—although it is still controversial—for Duke's Stage B cancer. When planning chemotherapy, your medical oncologist will consider many factors, including your age, the size and type of your tumor and its grade (aggressiveness), and the number of lymph nodes involved. Other indicators can include the results of many of the pathology studies of cell behavior.

When chemotherapy is used before surgery it is called neoadjuvant therapy. This is sometimes used in treating rectal cancer to shrink the tumor before surgery. When it is used after surgery to cure cancer or to keep it from spreading, it is called adjuvant therapy. The goal of adjuvant therapy is to protect against recurrence in patients with Duke's Stages B and C.

Although approximately 70 percent of patients who undergo resection surgery appear to be cured, about a third of them will eventually develop the disease again. So adjuvant chemotherapy reduces the chances of that happening. Adjuvant therapy is distinct from treating known metastatic disease with chemotherapy. Then it is called palliative chemotherapy, and the goal is to slow the spread of cancer and relieve pain.

Chemotherapy has long been associated with nausea, hair loss, and other difficult side effects, but these vary in intensity for each individual, and there are now medications that can help relieve some of these side effects.

Cytotoxic drugs—drugs used to kill cells—work in different ways. Flourouracil (5-FU) has been used alone to treat cancer or in combination with levamisole, or leucovorin. For colon cancer, chemotherapy is most commonly given by intravenous injection administered weekly in the oncologist's office, but this varies. For example, for Duke's Stage C cancer, chemotherapy with 5-FU and levamisole normally begins three to five weeks after surgery. This can vary in dosage amount, technique of administration, and length of time. 5-FU might be given intravenously daily for four weeks, then weekly for forty-eight weeks. Levamisole might be given orally for three days every two weeks for one year.

Until recently 5-FU combined with leucovorin was the mainstay of treatment for colorectal cancer. In 1996 Camptosar (CPT-11) was used alone in patients whose cancer recurred after treatment with 5-FU and leucovorin. In May 2000 the FDA approved the combination of Camptosar plus 5-FU and leucovorin for first-line therapy. In some patients this combination had better survival benefit than 5-FU and leucovorin. A third drug, called capecitabine (Xeloda), was approved in 2001 for metastatic colorectal cancer in specific groups of patients. Xeloda can be taken in pill form.

In August 2002, Eloxatin (oxaliplatin) was approved for use in combination with 5-FU in patients whose cancer did not respond to the combination of 5-FU and irinotecan. Other news drugs also are becoming available for use alone or in combination with 5-FU. Two drugs still in experimental stages are Tomudex and IMC-225.

Chemotherapy for Metastatic Colon Cancer

Fewer than half of colon cancer patients eventually develop metastatic disease either at a local or distant site. The treatment of any metastatic colon cancer requires focusing on the whole body, with the goal of easing the symptoms and halting progression of the disease for as long as possible to maintain a decent quality of life.

The liver is the most frequent site of metastatic colon cancer. Although isolated lesions can be surgically removed successfully from the liver, more widespread disease cannot. In that case, chemotherapy can be infused directly into the liver. Hepatic artery perfusion of chemotherapy has been used for a number of years with some success. Perfusion is a method of forcing a fluid through an organ via blood vessels, whereas infusion is the slow, continuous introduction of drugs into a vein.

Most of the blood flow to liver metastases comes from the hepatic artery, the main blood supply from the heart. Drugs can be administered through that artery via a port implanted in the body. This method has been successful in many cases.

Studies are under way to introduce anticancer drugs directly into the abdomen through a thin tube. This is intraperitoneal chemotherapy, and it is not yet in general use.

Immunotherapy

This treatment is designed to help the body's own immune system attack and destroy cancer cells. It uses agents made in a patient's own body or in the laboratory to direct the body's own defenses against disease. It is sometimes called biological response modifier (BRM). Side effects can vary widely but can include flulike symptoms such as fever, weakness, and chills, as well as nausea, vomiting, and diarrhea. A rash also can develop. This is being studied in several clinical trials, along with tumor vaccines and other approaches.

Clinical Trials

There are more than a hundred national clinical studies for treatment now in progress in the United States. These trials usually are carried out by university teaching hospitals, but the patients studied are scattered around the country, usually in comprehensive cancer centers or in other teaching hospitals. Your oncologist and the National Cancer Institute can tell you which clinical trials are available for colon cancer. If you qualify for any of the trials, you will be able to get the newest—and possibly best—treatment available. See the appendix for more information on clinical trials.

Follow-up Care

Periodic evaluations following treatment will help you find any recurrence of the disease early enough to treat it. However, there are no large-scale studies about how this affects mortality in the long term.

A review of the use of the tumor marker CEA suggests it is not a valuable screening test for colon cancer because of the large numbers of false positives and false negatives.

Recurrent Colon Cancer

If cancer recurs at a suture line it may be operable, especially if not enough was removed the first time. If it metastasizes to lungs or liver, these also may be surgically resected. In later stages, chemotherapy is used for pain relief.

Staying Healthy after Colon Cancer

It will take a while after surgery or chemotherapy to feel like walking to the corner, never mind running in a marathon, but do get moving as soon as possible. Exercise strengthens your heart and lungs and lifts your spirits. And ever more important to your recovery from colon cancer, it aids your digestion, helps eliminate gaseousness, and combined with balanced diet, will help keep your digestive system—and your colon—fit.

If you have a tendency to gain weight, watch your diet. Most people in America today eat twice as much as—if not more than—they need. This puts an enormous burden on your colon, not to mention the rest of your body. Make sure your diet includes plenty of fresh fruits and vegetables, because the fiber will help the digestive process. Avoid fats and sweets as they do just the opposite.

Clinical investigations suggest that diets high in total fat, protein, calories, alcohol, and meat, and low in calcium and folate, are associated with increased risk of colorectal cancer. Cereal fiber supplements and diet low in fat and high in fiber, fruits, and vegetables, however, do not reduce the rate of adenoma recurrent over a three- to four-year period.

Colon cancer rates are high in populations with high total fat intakes and lower in those consuming less fat. On average, fat makes up 40 to 45 percent of total caloric intake in high-incidence Western countries. In low-risk populations it accounts for only 10 percent of daily calories. A high-fat diet seems to increase bile acid secretion from the gallbladder. The potential mechanism of action of bile salts in colon cancer is unknown, but it has been suggested that it converts dietary substances to produce more bacteria.

Fiber is insoluble, such as wheat bran and cellulose, and soluble, usually dried beans. An increase in fiber potentially increases the fecal water, dilutes carcinogens, and decreases transit time.

Calcium

This appears to have some role in the regulation of the cells lining the colon, although it is not entirely clear how this works. Diets supplemented with calcium seem to minimize bile acids, and lab studies have suggested that calcium can inactivate carcinogens from fatty acids because it has an emulsyfing action, much the way detergent cuts the grease in a frying pan.

Aspirin and Other Anti-inflammatory Drugs (NSAIDs)

These also are said to reduce deaths from colon cancer, but only in the earliest stages, according to current research. It is believed to stop the growth of polyps in the colon that might become aggressive over time. It might be aspirin's ability to block production of prostaglandins, certain fatty acids, that might regulate the growth of cells. Many studies show that regular aspirin users have less colon cancer. In 2003 the most recent study, by the University of North Carolina and Dartmouth College and Hitchcock Medical Center, was reported in the *New England Journal of Medicine*. One aspirin every other day for twenty years is said to cut the risk in half. Some doctors routinely recommend aspirin to patients over fifty to cut the risk of heart disease, an already established benefit. However, aspirin in certain people can cause blood loss that will appear in the stool. Ask your doctor about this.

Exercise

A sedentary lifestyle has been associated in nearly all studies with an increased risk of colon cancer. You can cut your risk in half with exercise. The only question in the studies is whether the exercise alone, or combined with better diet, is responsible. Obesity doubles the risk in premenopausal women.

Here are some general rules for preventing colon cancer:

- Have a digital rectal exam and a fecal occult blood test annually.
- Have a sigmoidoscopy every five years, or a colonoscopy or double-contrast barium enema every five to ten years. Have all noncancerous polyps removed to help prevent colorectal cancer before it starts.
- If you or a family member has a history of colon cancer; benign colorectal polyps; inflammatory bowel disease; or breast, ovarian, or endometrial cancer, talk to your doctor about early screening.

- Eat a diet rich in fruits and vegetables and whole grains and low in fat.
- Eat foods with folate such as leafy green vegetables—or take a daily multivitamin containing 0.4 microgram of folic acid.
- If you drink alcohol, do so in moderation.
- Do not smoke. It is associated with an increased tendency to form polyps.
- Exercise for at least twenty minutes three to four days a week.

Anorectal and Perianal Disorders

The most common anal and perianal diseases are hemorrhoids, anal fissures, fistulas, pilonidal sinus diseases, and perianal skin conditions. Most of these conditions cause bleeding, pain, swelling, discharge, and itching. Many people are embarrassed to talk with their physicians in detail about such conditions, and as a result sometimes they are not examined or diagnosed properly. Many anorectal or perianal diseases are often secondary to more serious gastrointestinal conditions or sexually transmitted diseases. If the core problem is addressed, the anal problems can be treated effectively. Also, if these conditions are not treated, they can lead to serious complications and more complicated treatment. A proper analysis of any chronic condition of the anal area means more than just a digital exam. It should include at the very least an endoscopic examination of the rectum.

Hemorrhoids

Hemorrhoids are so common that it is believed up to half the population has them by age fifty. Hemorrhoids are enlarged, painful veins in the rectum that can develop from two different places. There are two sets of veins that drain the blood from the lower rectum and anus. The internal veins can become swollen to form internal hemorrhoids. Unless they are severe, these cannot be seen or felt. Hemorrhoids from swollen external veins can be seen and felt around the outside of the anus. External hemorrhoids, when thrombosed, can be very painful. A blood clot occurs in a hemorrhoid, causing it to become even more swollen and painful. Pain is usually worse at bowel movements or sometimes with sitting.

Hemorrhoids are associated with constipation and straining at bowel movements as well as pregnancy because these conditions are believed to increase pressure in the hemorrhoid veins, thus causing them to swell. Liver disease also can cause increased pressure in the veins.

When internal hemorrhoids swell and extend through the anus they are prolapsed. Sometimes they can gently be pushed back to solve the problem. If the hemorrhoids cannot be pushed back, they may swell more and become trapped outside the anus and require medical care. Prolapsed hemorrhoids can lead to an itching in the anus called pruritus ani.

Symptoms of Hemorrhoids

The most common complaint from internal hemorrhoids is painless bleeding. Bright red blood can be seen on the outside of the stool, on the toilet paper, or dripping into the toilet. This usually doesn't last long. Any rectal bleeding needs to be taken seriously because it may not always be caused by hemorrhoids. Inflammatory bowel disease and colorectal cancer can cause such bleeding. It is important to see your doctor if you develop bleeding between bowel movements or if you are over forty or have a family history of colon cancer.

At forty-two, Phil was concerned about rectal bleeding because his father had died from colon cancer. The bleeding, Phil said, occurred for six days and did not contain clots. It showed up on the surface of the bowel movement and in the water in the bowl as well as on the paper. His anal area was somewhat sore, but he didn't feel anything out of the ordinary. However, he admitted to being more constipated than usual during the past month. A colonoscopy revealed that Phil had internal hemorrhoids coated with fresh blood, but no other lesions were found. He was given a high-fiber diet and told to drink at least six glassfuls of water a day. He also was prescribed a steroid suppository for two weeks and told to wipe with moisturized pads to relieve irritation.

There may be times when you need to get emergency care. If you have significant bleeding and pain and you can't reach your doctor, go to the emergency room at a hospital.

Self-Care for Hemorrhoids

Many creams, ointments, and suppositories are sold as pain relievers and medicines for hemorrhoids. They are of little help and sometimes might even cause the hemorrhoids to take longer to heal. Ask your doctor before you use any of these.

Avoid sitting for long periods of time, or sit on an air doughnut. A sitz bath three times a day and after each bowel movement can relieve the pain and swelling of hemorrhoids. Sit in the bath for at least fifteen minutes. Be sure to dry the area thoroughly.

Drink more fluids and eat more leafy green vegetables. This makes stools bulkier and softer to relieve constipation. Be cautious about taking over-the-counter stool softeners and laxatives.

Medical Treatment for Hemorrhoids

For a painful thrombosed hemorrhoid that cannot be relieved with self-care, ask your doctor about having the clot removed. Anesthetic is used to numb the area, and a small cut in the hemorrhoid will remove the clot. Follow up with sitz baths at home and frequent change of dressings.

Hemorrhoids can be injected with a medication to shrink them, or small rubber bands can be placed around them to cut off the blood supply so they die. These procedures usually can be done in the doctor's office and don't require general anesthesia.

Less common treatments include cryotherapy to freeze the hemorrhoid off, or laser therapy to burn it off. A prolapsed internal hemorrhoid that cannot be reduced or pushed back may require surgery. Sometimes it is necessary for a surgeon to cut off the hemorrhoids. In this case, general anesthesia or a spinal anesthetic is used.

Anal Fissures

An anal fissure is a painful tear or crack in the anal canal that is probably caused by trauma from the passage of a hard or painful bowel movement. A tear can involve only the mucous lining, but over time may go deeper into the anal lining. Minor tears heal rapidly, but if there are underlying abnormalities of the internal sphincter, such tears progress to acute and chronic fissures. The area becomes so raw and stretched that any bowel movement is painful and creates fear and anxiety. There is no significant bleeding from anal fissures, but most people also report bright red blood on the stool.

Anal fissures tend to occur in young and middle-aged men more than women and also in people who have had previous anal surgery and the associated scarring.

Treatment must break the cycle of constipation with fiber supplementation and stool laxatives as needed. Mineral oil may facilitate passage of bowel movements without as much stretching or abrasion of the anal mucosa. Sitz baths relieve pain. However, if the high-fiber diet is abandoned, the fissures recur in as many as 70 percent of cases.

Topical medication such as NTG ointment (nitroglycerin) applied to the fissure is thought to relax the sphincter and help relieve some of the pain associated with sphincter spasm. However, use of this ointment is still controversial because of adverse side effects, including headache and dizziness.

Botox (botulism toxin) injected directly into the sphincter is a newer therapy. This is like a sphincterectomy without surgery, but symptoms often return. Acute anal fissures that remain symptomatic for three to four months usually need surgery. Sphincterectomy is performed with general anesthesia. The internal sphincter is cut to relieve the tension so the fissure can heal.

Fistula in Ano

A fistula in ano is nearly always caused by a previous anorectal abscess. Anal canal glands offer a pathway for infecting organisms to reach the intramuscular spaces. The infection begins in the anal gland and progresses into the muscular wall of the anal sphincters to cause an abscess.

People who get these fistulas may have inflammatory bowel disease, diverticulitis, HIV infection, or previous radiation therapy for prostate or rectal cancer. Men are twice as vulnerable as women to this condition which usually occurs in the thirties.

Symptoms include perianal discharge, pain, swelling, bleeding, diarrhea, and skin excoriation. A change in bowel habits and weight loss also are symptoms.

Correct diagnosis can be made with a fistulography, the injection of a contrast dye through the internal opening followed by X-rays. Anal ultrasound, MRI, CT scan, and barium enema also are sometime used in diagnosis. Anal manometry can help evaluate the pressure exerted by the sphincter.

There is no ideal medical treatment, but surgery—fistulotomy—is used to repair it.

Pilonidal Cyst

A pilonial cyst occurs at the bottom of the tailbone and can become infected and filled with pus. It is technically called a pilonidal abscess and looks like a large pimple at the bottom of the tailbone, just above the crack of the buttocks. Most doctors believe that pilonidal cysts are caused by ingrown hairs. Pilonidal means "nest of hair." It is common to find hair follicles inside the cyst. It is more common in young men than in women.

Pilonidal cysts are thought to be acquired through trauma to the base of the spine. During World War II, more than eighty thousand soldiers developed pilonidal cysts that required them to be hospitalized. The cysts were caused by irritation from riding in bumpy jeeps. For a while it was actually called "jeep disease."

Symptoms include pain, swelling, and redness at the bottom of the spine; draining pus; and fever. A pilonidal cyst is an abscess or boil, and, like other boils, it does not get better with antibiotics. It needs to be drained or lanced.

There are several ways by which a pilonidal cyst can be treated:

1. The doctor will make an incision to drain the cyst, remove the hair follicles, and pack the cavity with gauze, which will need to be changed often. This simple procedure can be done in the doctor's office.

2. To avoid the gauze dressing, the cavity could also be stitched. This technique requires outpatient surgery and a physician trained in the procedure. It takes about six weeks to heal.

3. Immediate closing of the wound is another option, but there is a high chance that the cyst will grow back. This is also done with local anesthetic as outpatient surgery.

Proctitis

Proctitis is an inflammation of the anus and lining of the lower part—the last six inches—of the rectum. It can be a temporary condition or it can become chronic and last for weeks or months. The most common cause of proctitis is sexually transmitted diseases in homosexual men and people who engage in anal intercourse with many partners. However, it also can be caused by infections such as herpes simplex, anal warts (HPV), ulcerative colitis, or Crohn's disease (IBD); physical agents such as chemicals or foreign objects; trauma; or having had radiation or treatment with antibiotics.

Symptoms of proctitis can vary greatly, from minor irritation to bleeding and discharge. Symptoms include:

- Pain during a bowel movement
- Soreness in the anal and rectal area
- Feeling that bowels are not empty after a movement
- Involuntary spasms and cramping during bowel movements
- Bleeding and discharge

Diagnosis and treatment of proctitis depend on the cause. If STDs are involved, they have to be correctly diagnosed and treated. If it is caused by inflammatory bowel disease, that must be treated (see chapter 10). In any case an endoscopic examination of the rectum and a biopsy should be done.

In most cases proctitis goes away with treatment. If the disease comes from a chronic illness, surgery may be required. If it stems from ulcerative colitis, it may flare up now and then. And surgery may be needed to remove the diseased part of the GI tract. If proctitis goes untreated, it may result in severe bleeding, anemia, and fistulas, which can occur in many parts of the body. Fistulas connect the rectum to the skin, and feces may come out of an opening other than the anus. Fistulas also become infected and cause even more complications.

Pruritus Ani

Pruritus ani is an unpleasant sensation that creates an irresistible urge to scratch the anus. It can occur anytime but usually after a bowel movement or before falling asleep. The skin around the anus may be inflamed and in some cases cracked and bleeding. In chronic cases, the anal ring may have a shiny appearance. It affects about 5 percent of the population, men more than women, and most commonly people in their forties through sixties.

Pruritus ani usually is caused by other conditions such as infections, psoriasis, or gastrointestinal problems such as prolapsed hemorrhoids. When these conditions are treated, the disease usually abates.

Problems keeping the anal area dry, or the use of irritants including powders, creams, and soaps, also may contribute to the cause. Obese people, for example, cannot adequately dry the anal area, and itching results. A digital rectal exam allows the doctor to look for secondary causes, such as a local malignancy.

Most creams and ointments found in the drugstore for anal itching are not effective. Some that may provide relief include Anusol ointment and Anusol-HC ointment. Hydroxyzine and chlorpheniramine are designed for pruritis and are sedatives to help break the cycle of scratching during sleep. Systemic antihistamines may be helpful, especially to people who scratch at night. Cotton gloves worn at night may help prevent damage from unconscious scratching.

If conservative measures don't help in a few weeks, then your doctor needs to do some more investigations. Diet needs to be considered, too. Eating spicy or acidic foods can often cause anal itching, so eliminating them from the diet may help.

Benign and Malignant Anal Tumors

A variety of tumors, both benign and malignant, may affect the anal area. There is a wide variation of epithelial tissue in the anal canal that gives rise to tumors. However, these tumors represent only a small portion of the tumors in the colorectal area.

Homosexual men are at high risk for anal tumors, but they also can be caused by chronic inflammatory disease of the anal region such as perianal Crohn's disease, previous pelvic radiation, and chronic fistula disease. Anal cancer is uncommon, but usually is curable depending on location, size, and how aggressive the cancer cells are.

The most common symptoms are rectal bleeding, deep anal pain, discharge of mucus, incontinence, and the feeling of a mass in the anal region.

Malignant anal tumors are treated with combined chemotherapy and radiation. This treatment is usually successful; if not, surgery is required. Part of the sphincter can be removed without damaging fecal control.

Rectal Prolapse

When a layer of rectal tissue slides through the anal opening, it is a rectal prolapse. It may begin with an internal prolapse of the rectal wall and progress to a full prolapse. Half of all prolapses are caused by chronic bowel straining because of constipation. Weakness of the pelvic floor and low pressure in the resting sphincter also are associated with prolapse. It can be caused by benign prostatic hypertrophy, chronic obstructive pulmonary disease, cystic fibrosis, whooping cough, spinal problems, parasitic infections, and neurological disorders such as multiple sclerosis.

Rectal prolapse is more common with people over sixty-five and affects about ten people per thousand in the population. Six times more women than men have the condition. It leads to increasing difficulties with rectal bleeding, ulceration, and incontinence. In rare cases it can lead to strangulation of the rectal tissue, which cuts off the blood supply and can lead to gangrene.

In general, a prolapse can be reduced with gentle digital pressure using sedation and local anesthesia. The contributing factors, such as constipation, need to be treated. If the prolapse is more complicated, it may need to be surgically repaired.

Rectal Pain

Rectal pain is a common problem, and everybody has experienced it at one time or another. Usually it appears as a mild irritation, but sometimes the pain is severe enough to be incapacitating. Most of the conditions that cause rectal pain, such as hemorrhoids and anal fissures, are not serious. There are less likely reasons for rectal pain, including cancer, and infections such as anorectal abscesses or proctitis.

Proctalgia Fugax

This is fleeting rectal pain and occurs in about 8 percent of Americans, more commonly in women and in people younger than forty-five. The cause is unknown, but most doctors believe it is a result of a spasm of the anal sphincter muscle. Although the pain lasts less than a minute, it is sudden and intense. However, in some cases the spasm can continue for an hour. It is a sharp, stabbing, or cramplike pain at the anal opening, and it can wake someone from a sound sleep. Attacks seem to occur in clusters, happening daily for a while, then going away for months or weeks.

Levator Ani Syndrome

This also occurs in women more than men and affects 6 percent of the population. Levator ani refers to the group of muscles that surrounds and supports the anus. Spasms of these muscles are believed to cause rectal pain, a tight pressure high inside the rectal passage. The sensation lasts for about twenty minutes and tends to recur at regular intervals. It is made worse by sitting and improves with walking or standing.

A digital rectal exam can diagnose this condition. You can stop the pain by sitting in a tub of hot water and massaging the levator ani muscles to relieve the spasm. Over-the-counter anti-inflammatory medications such as ibuprofen or naproxen may relieve pain.

Any continuing pain or signs of bleeding need to be diagnosed by a doctor.

Chapter 11

The Abdominal Cavity

THE ABDOMINAL CAVITY is the largest hollow space in your body. The area is between the diaphragm and the top of your pelvic cavity and is surrounded by the spine and the abdominal and other muscles. This cavity contains the lower part of the esophagus, the stomach, small intestine, colon, rectum, gallbladder, liver, pancreas, spleen, kidneys, and bladder. The abdominal cavity's inside wall is lined with a membrane called the peritoneum. This membrane also lines each organ or structure in the cavity. This is the visceral peritoneum. Various things can go wrong in the cavity, such as sections of gut becoming herniated, the space can fill with fluid, and infections can occur. Conditions occurring within the cavity include:

- Inguinal, femoral, ventral, and umbilical hernia
- Hiatal hernia
- Appendicitis

Abdominal Wall and Groin Hernias

When a part of the intestine bulges through a weak area of muscle in the abdominal wall or through a sphincter opening, it causes a hernia. Most hernias occur because of increased abdominal pressure from obesity, pregnancy, chronic cough, constipation, heavy lifting, bladder obstruction, or when fluid accumulates in the peritoneal cavity. Some hernias are painful, some are not. There are three primary types of abdominal hernias: groin, umbilical, and hiatal.

Groin Hernias

Sam, thirty-five, was carrying furniture out to a moving van in preparation for his family's move to a new home. When he strained to pick up a particularly heavy coffee table, he suddenly felt a sharp pain in his right groin. Later he noticed that a painful bulge had developed in his groin, but it disappeared when he lay on his back. Sam didn't like going to a doctor, so he ignored the condition. After several months, the pain and the bulge increased and he finally went to a doctor. With the history and physical findings, the doctor diagnosed an indirect inguinal hernia and scheduled Sam for surgery. The hernia was repaired successfully, and Sam went home from the hospital in a few days.

People don't always know when they get a hernia. Sometimes they feel them. They may get a painful or painless lump that may change with position.

Inguinal Hernia

This occurs in the groin, the area between the abdomen and the thigh. Intestines push through a weak spot in the inguinal canal. This is a triangle-shaped opening (Hesselbach's triangle) between layers of abdominal muscles near the groin. A hernia is not always visible, but usually you feel it. A lump in the groin near the thigh is an obvious symptom of hernia, as is pain in the groin. In severe cases, a hernia can partially or completely block the intestine. If a loop of bowel becomes trapped in the hernia (strangulated), the bowel will be obstructed or it can lose its blood supply. Both conditions, although rare, can be life-threatening.

An indirect inguinal hernia is the herniation of abdominal contents through the internal ring. This is more likely to strangulate, which often occurs without warning. It is the most common type of hernia in men and women.

Femoral Hernia

This also occurs in the groin area, but it develops lower than the inguinal hernia at or very near the leg crease. Often it is hard to differentiate clinically between the two, but finding a painful lump or bulge on the leg crease adjacent to the pubic area suggests a femoral hernia. Sometimes you can get both an inguinal and a femoral hernia.

The defect itself occurs in an anatomic triangular-shaped "gap" among the following three structures: the inguinal ligament (a tendinous cord that creates the leg crease), the lower side of the pubic bone, and the femoral vein (major vein of the leg). This gap is somewhat larger in women because of the shape and angle of the pelvis. When an acutely painful lump or bulge is found on the leg crease adjacent to the pubic area, it suggests a femoral hernia.

Abdominal contents can herniate through the femoral sheath, which contains the nerve, artery, vein, lymphatics, extra space—and the hernia occurs.

Because of the shape of their pelvis, women get femoral hernias five times more often than men, and it is most common in thin, elderly women.

An inguinal or femoral hernia is fairly easy to diagnose with a physical exam, X-rays, and blood tests to check for blockage of the intestine. However, your doctor must also rule out other possible causes, including an enlarged lymph node, femoral aneurysm, psoas abscess, or ectopic testes in a man. A hernia is most often confused with a swollen lymph node.

Repairing Hernias Surgically

Nearly a hundred thousand hernia repairs are performed each year in the United States. Many are done with conventional open surgery, and some are performed laparoscopically. The main treatment for inguinal hernia is surgery to repair the opening in the muscle wall. This surgery is called herniorrhaphy. Sometimes the weak area is reinforced with steel mesh or wire, which is more effective than sutures. This operation is called hernioplasty. If the protruding intestine becomes twisted or traps fecal matter, part of the intestine might need to be removed. This is called a bowel resection.

Laparoscopic surgery is becoming a common way to repair a hernia. Three small incisions are made in the abdominal wall: one for the laparoscope and the other two for surgical instruments. Under the guidance of video camera attached to the laparoscope, a strong, flexible patch is stapled in place over the defect in the abdominal wall.

Inguinal hernia repair is the most frequently performed operation in general surgery. The standard method for inguinal hernia repair changed little over a hundred years until the introduction of synthetic mesh. The mesh can be placed by using either an open approach or laparoscopic surgery. Laparoscopic surgery is now popular.

Compared with conventional open surgery, the laparoscopic technique results in more rapid recovery, fewer surgical wound infections, and reduced recurrence. It reduces recovery time and the need for postoperative anesthesia compared with open repair.

Ventral Hernia

A ventral hernia usually arises in the abdominal wall where a previous surgical incision was made. The abdominal muscles have weakened, and this leads to a bulge or tear. The inner lining of the abdomen pushes through the weakened area of the abdomen to form a sac. Ventral hernias also can develop at the navel or other areas and will not go away by themselves.

Umbilical Hernia

An umbilical hernia is a protrusion of the peritoneum and fluid, or a portion of abdominal organs through the umbilical ring—the fibrous and muscle tissue around the navel. An infant may get such a hernia when the umbilical ring or muscle doesn't close properly. This ring is where the umbilical blood vessels passed to provide nourishment to the developing fetus. This hernia creates an "outie" rather than an "innie" at the navel.

The hernia, usually painless, appears as a soft swelling beneath the skin that often protrudes when the baby is upright, or with crying or straining. The area of the hernia can vary from less than a centimeter to more than five in diameter. Small hernias close spontaneously by the time the baby is three or four, but those that do not close may need surgery. Umbilical hernias are quite common in babies and may be as high as one in six. They tend to occur slightly more often in African American infants.

Although most common in infants, umbilical hernias can occur later in life.

Hiatal Hernia

When the upper part of the stomach pushes through the esophageal hiatus, an opening in the diaphragm, the muscle that separates the abdomen from the chest, it results in a hiatal hernia.

After food travels through the esophagus it passes through an opening called the esophageal hiatus to enter the stomach. At the bottom of the esophagus, the lower esophageal sphincter (LES) acts as a valve (see chapter 4). The hiatus acts like a second valve. Normally the hiatus and the LES line up with each other to keep stomach contents from backing up or refluxing into the esophagus. But the hiatus can stretch because of muscle weakness or too much abdominal pressure. When this occurs, the stomach can slip through the hiatus, causing a hiatal hernia. A hiatal hernia usually is detected when someone gets X-rays or endoscopic tests for heartburn or reflux disease.

Sliding Hernias   These are the most common. About half of people over fifty have one. These hernias usually don't cause problems, but they are associated with reflux. If the hernia is associated with significant reflux symptoms that cause difficulty breathing or bleeding, it needs to be surgically repaired.

Paraesophageal Hernias   These are less common than the sliding type, but they are more dangerous. In this case, the esophagus remains where it is but the stomach moves up through the opening in the hiatus and into the chest. When this rolling movement of the stomach into the chest happens, it puts the stomach at risk for twisting in the chest (volvulus). This causes an obstruction that can be life-threatening. Once a paraesophageal hernia has been diagnosed it should be surgically corrected, even if it causes no symptoms.

Most hiatal hernias are not too bothersome, and many people over age fifty have them. Some people do get heartburn from gastric reflux and may need drug therapy. If the hernia is in danger of becoming twisted and cutting off the blood supply to the stomach, the hernia would need to be repaired. Usually there are ample symptoms to bring this complication to medical attention.

Of the several different types of hiatal hernias, some may include a Richter component, which means part of the wall of the intestine is engaged in the hernia sac. This does not affect the passage of bowel contents, so even though there is strangulation, there is no obstruction. Obstruction does not occur with these types of hernias, but strangulation and perforation may, so they must be repaired.

Easing the Discomfort of a Hiatal Hernia

When a hiatal hernia doesn't cause pain or too much discomfort, nothing needs to be done about it. But if it does cause symptoms, here are ways to ease the discomfort:

- Work with your doctor to treat heartburn or reflux disease with diet and medication.
- Avoid spicy and fatty foods that may cause symptoms.
- Eat smaller, more frequent meals.
- Avoid lying down for three hours after eating.
- Raise the head of your bed four to eight inches.
- Avoid wearing tight clothing around your waist.

Other Treatment of a Hiatal Hernia

When a hiatal hernia is associated with reflux disease, treatment must focus on clearing up that condition (see chapter 4). Surgery may be required if the GERD does not respond to treatment and the hernia is at risk of twisting. This could cut off the blood supply, a serious complication.

Conventional or laparoscopic surgery can be used to repair the hiatal hernia. In recent years, laparoscopic herniorrhaphy has become a widely accepted surgical treatment. The technique allows the surgeon to pull the sac of the hernia down out of the chest and repair the hole in the diaphragm. After the repair of the hernia defect, fundoplication can be performed if needed. In this operation the fundus of the stomach, on the left of the esophagus and main portion of the stomach, is wrapped around the back of the esophagus until it is once again in front of this structure. The portion of the fundus that is now on the right side of the esophagus is sutured to the portion on the left side to keep the wrap in place. The fundoplication resembles a buttoned shirt collar. The collar is the fundus wrap, and the neck represents the esophagus imbricated into the wrap. This creates a security valve in the esophagus that won't allow the stomach to go up into the chest.

Preventing Abdominal Hernias

Abdominal hernias can happen when you are out of shape and suddenly do strenuous activity involving abdominal muscles or if you are overweight and putting pressure on those muscles. Sudden physical exertion such as weight lifting or doing sit-ups improperly can do it. Hernias also can be caused by coughing or straining to move your bowels. Tight clothing around the waist will aggravate a hiatal hernia, as will eating foods that cause gastric reflux. Some general commonsense rules can help you avoid abdominal hernias:

- Maintain good body weight so you are not putting undo strain on your abdominal muscles.
- When you lift heavy objects, use your legs for leverage, not your back and abdomen.
- Don't sit up from a prone position on your back without first bending your knees.

Appendicitis

You don't really need your appendix, and if you are one of the many people who had it removed in childhood, you already know that. This little worm-shaped pouch that hangs from the cecum, the beginning of the colon, may be useless, but it can cause a great deal of pain and a medical emergency if it gets infected. Left untreated, an infected appendix can burst and spread infection into the abdominal cavity. Appendicitis can happen at any age but most often occurs between ages ten and thirty. It's probably the most common reason for surgery for children. Anyone with symptoms needs to get to a doctor immediately, within twelve hours if possible. There are about 250,000 new cases per year in the United States.

Appendicitis is generally caused by obstruction of the appendix by an appendicolith—or stone. This obstruction, which may be a collection of debris from the colon, leads to pressure buildup, bacterial invasion, and increased inflammation. Perforation follows if it is not treated, and this leads to peritonitis, a potentially fatal infection of the peritoneum—the membrane around the abdominal organs.

Symptoms of Appendicitis

Symptoms of appendicitis are often variable, and this can impede an easy diagnosis. Usually there are three stages of appendicitis: the edematous stage; the purulent stage, when the appendix has perforated; and the gangrenous stage, when peritonitis is present. The first sign of appendicitis usually is a colicky type of abdominal pain that may be accompanied by diarrhea. The pain may begin in the middle of the abdomen, then migrate to the lower right side. The pain becomes worse when you move, take deep breaths, cough, or sneeze. Nausea and vomiting may follow. Some people get flushed from a body temperature increase, may feel breathless, and have an offensive smell on their breath. One clue that it may be appendicitis rather than another abdominal infection is that abdominal pain begins *before* nausea and vomiting, rather than after. However, these typical pain patterns are present in only 20 percent of people.

The location of pain is completely dependent on the position of the appendix. For example, if you have an elevated cecum (riding high in the abdominal cavity), your pain will be higher up.

If the appendix is irritating the bladder, symptoms of a bladder infection, such as feeling an increased need to urinate, may occur. In women the pain also could be associated with inflammation of the ovaries or fallopian tubes. In addition, appendicitis can mimic pelvic inflammatory disease.

In some people, the appendix sticks out in an unusual place or at an odd angle. In these cases, appendicitis can cause other symptoms such as pain in the sides or the back, pain during urinating, or pain in the upper left side of the abdomen.

Jane woke up one morning not feeling quite right. She ate breakfast and went to work. By noon she had a dull, achy pain just above her navel that caused her to skip eating lunch. The pain became worse in the afternoon, so she left work early. After a bowl of soup for dinner, she went to bed but could not sleep well because of the discomfort and feeling of nausea. She took a sleeping pill, but that didn't help. When the doctor pressed on the lower right part of her abdomen, it hurt Jane. It also made her feel nauseous.

If you suspect appendicitis, get to a doctor or a hospital quickly. Don't take any pain medications that can mask the symptoms because the doctor needs to know about the pain. In most people the site of the pain is tender to the touch. Don't take remedies to relieve diarrhea or constipation either, because these can cause the appendix to burst.

Diagnosis of Appendicitis

Because appendicitis symptoms vary and can be confused with many other conditions, it's critical that you get a medical diagnosis as soon as possible. High suspicion is critical to avoid missing a diagnosis of appendicitis. Because doctors tend to err on the side of caution, in three out of ten cases, a perfectly sound appendix is removed.

A medical history is crucial along with a careful physical examination. By pressing on the lower right part of the abdomen and sometimes by doing a digital rectal exam to exclude other causes of pain, doctors can determine if it is appendicitis. Sometimes women may get a gynecological exam to rule out other possible causes of pain in the area.

Some diagnostic tests also are needed. Ultrasound can detect a calcified stone in the appendix area. If ultrasound is negative or inconclusive but clinical suspicion is high, a CT scan may confirm the diagnosis by visualizing inflammation. Blood tests check for signs of infection, such as a high white blood cell count. Urine tests rule out urinary tract infection.

Because the symptoms are so variable, other possible causes of the pain must be ruled out. These include Crohn's disease, pelvic abscess, ovarian or fallopian tube disease, pelvic inflammatory disease, gallbladder inflammation, or intestinal perforation due to obstruction such as right-side colon cancer.

Special Concerns During pregnancy the appendix moves to another position to make way for the growing fetus. Although nausea, vomiting, and anorexia are common early in a pregnancy, when these occur later, it could be appendicitis. It is possible to have an appendectomy during pregnancy, but it puts the mother and child at more risk.

Women of childbearing age with appendicitis are misdiagnosed at least a third of the time because symptoms are similar to those of pelvic inflammatory disease (PID), gastroenteritis, or urinary tract infections.

Children are misdiagnosed 25 to 30 percent of the time. The appendicitis is most commonly blamed on gastroenteritis or upper respiratory infection. Misdiagnosis also is increased in the elderly, who may have many other medical conditions.

Removing the Appendix

If the appendix is infected, it must come out. People with equivocal signs of the condition may be watched and sometimes treated with antibiotics. In the past, appendectomy required open abdominal surgery, general anesthesia, and a long hospital stay. Unless there are complications, doctors now use laparoscopic surgery. Making several tiny cuts in the lower right abdomen, the surgeon can insert a miniature camera and surgical instruments and remove the appendix. Laparoscopic surgery has reduced the risk of wound infection and requires less recuperative time.

Fluid management is the intravenous administration of salt and water to make up for bodily losses. This is critical following surgery, and antibiotic therapy is necessary to prevent infection. Antibiotics are designed to cover anerobic bacteria causing an infection.

In uncomplicated cases, a two- to three-day hospital stay is typical. Most patients go home when their temperature is normal and the bowel begins to function again. The stitches are removed in ten days, and within four to six weeks, normal life resumes.

About a fifth of the patients who undergo surgery already have a ruptured appendix and peritonitis has begun. This is inflammation of the peritoneum, the membrane around the internal organs. Treatment with antibiotics helps make this less risky. But there still is risk of an abscess forming in the abdominal cavity, and that would require draining. Usually this can be accomplished by an interventional radiologist putting a catheter in the abdomen under X-ray guidance.

In a few cases, adhesions from scar tissue may develop within three months of surgery and block or obstruct the bowel; this may require emergency surgery.

PART III

Maintaining Gastrointestinal Health

Chapter 12

A Commonsense Guide to Diet and Exercise

IF EVERYONE IN THE WORLD ate properly, exercised regularly, got regular checkups and screenings—and did not smoke—many doctors would be out of work. Throughout this book we've talked about steps you can take to lower your risk factors for many gastrointestinal diseases. Here are some reminders along with guidelines for screening to avoid illness. There's also a section on preventing gastroenteritis when you travel.

Diet and Nutrition

A well-balanced nutritious diet of protein, fruits and vegetables, whole grains, and a small amount of unsaturated fat, is the best way to maintain health. Fiber in the form of cereals, whole grains, and fresh fruits and vegetables helps flush the fats and waste products from the body with more efficiency. When there is no fiber to transport the waste matter through the colon and out of the body, it stays in the colon, where it may contribute to the growth of polyps. These polyps, if undiscovered, can become cancerous.

If you have a preexisting condition such as ulcers or esophagitis, avoid spicy foods, which may stimulate acid secretion and aggravate the lining of the digestive tract. Among the worst offenders are black pepper, chili pepper, and some curries.

Small amounts of fat are necessary, but too much will force the gallbladder to work too hard, and stimulate the pancreas enough to cause pain. High-fat diets tend to relax the lower esophageal sphincter and allow gastrointestinal reflux.

Saturated fat should account for only 10 percent and total fat 30 percent or less. Saturated fat elevates your cholesterol. Dietary fats from unsaturated fats such as olive oil, corn oil, and fish oils are the best kinds.

Fat is more concentrated than other calories. There are twice as many calories in a gram of fat than there are in a gram of any other kind of food.

Drink Plenty of Water

Half of your body is water, and it needs replenishing. Although we get a certain amount of water in our foods, especially produce, we need to drink eight glassfuls a day or about two quarts. The fiber we eat absorbs water from our body. Few people drink enough water, relying mostly on soft drinks, juices, or coffee and tea. Caffeinated drinks actually dehydrate your body. Sufficient water will help avoid constipation and any number of other problems.

Exercise

Even moderate exercise such as a daily long walk brings oxygen into your digestive system and helps it do its job. Exercise helps control appetite. Exercise increases your metabolism so you burn calories. It stabilizes insulin and blood sugar so you don't feel hungry. It reduces stress, which is a causative factor in irritable bowel syndrome and some other conditions. Constipation, more common in women, is frequently felt to be caused by a sedentary lifestyle. Exercise promotes laxation, which in turn relieves constipation. Exercise is critical to bring oxygen to your digestive system and keep the process going, especially through the lower intestinal tract.

The best exercises for the gastrointestinal system are swimming, walking, and cycling. It doesn't matter what type you do, as long as you do it consistently.

Stay in Shape

Being overweight is not only risky for heart disease and cancer, it also adds to and causes gastrointestinal problems such as gallbladder disease and fatty liver. The best way to lose weight is to cut calories and increase activity. If you find it difficult, ask your doctor for a medical program that works, or sign up with Weight Watchers, a medically sound program that works. Ask your doctor for help. The American Gastroenterology Association has declared that all of its member physicians should help their overweight patients get in shape. Learn all you can about good nutrition and let common sense be your guide.

Don't Smoke

Smoking, of course, cuts off the oxygen in your body and is a huge contributor to digestive problems and cancers. Smoking increases your risk of acid reflux disease as well as esophageal cancer, stomach cancer, and ulcers. These conditions are especially high among smokers, as are cancers of the entire upper digestive tract. You may think the smoke is going only to your lungs, but it is contaminating the upper part of your digestive tract as well—including your mouth.

Alcohol in Moderation

Alcohol is good in moderation and bad in excess. It is the dietary factor most associated with gastrointestinal illness. It can damage the entire digestive tract and cause chronic liver problems. Excess alcohol is directly responsible for cancer of the esophagus, bleeding of the stomach lining, ulcers, and destruction of the pancreas and liver.

Screening for Prevention

Colon Cancer

Everyone fifty or over should be screened for colorectal cancer with an annual fecal occult blood test and a sigmoidoscopy or colonoscopy every few years. There is no set interval between these tests, but if you have had cancer or have a family history of colon cancer, or if you have inflammatory bowel disease, or rectal bleeding or polyps, you should have a colonoscopy more often. Remember, colon cancer always begins with a polyp. Therefore, if polyps are found early and removed, you may avoid getting colon cancer. People at risk should get a colonoscopy every three to five years. Ask you doctor about this.

Upper GI Endoscopy

Some people feel that perhaps they should have an endoscopic examination of their upper gastrointestinal tract after middle age. Generally this is not necessary unless you have symptoms, or if you are Japanese and at risk for problems in the upper digestive tract.

Viral Hepatitis

Screening and/or vaccination for hepatitis B is recommended for all pregnant women and others at high risk for this disease, such as day-care workers and travelers.

Celiac Disease

If you have a family history of celiac disease, you should be screened for this.

Preventing Gastrointestinal Problems
When You Travel

There is a rapid and dramatic change in the type of organisms your gastrointestinal system encounters when you go from an industrialized country to a developing country. The new organisms often overcome your system's defense mechanisms. Americans make 250 million trips to other countries each year. Ten million of them are to developing countries, and 60 percent of travelers become ill as a result of their travels. This is according to research by emergency physicians.

Before you go abroad, always check with your doctor to see if you need vaccinations against viral hepatitis or any other disease.

Travelers' Gastroenteritis

Travelers' diarrhea affects 20 to 50 percent of tourists, usually within the first week of travel, although they can occur later, even after you return home. Attacks begin abruptly with bloating, cramps, and nausea. Usually it is acute and resolves within seven days. It lasts from three to four days, and about 10 percent of cases last a week. In some people diarrhea is accompanied by vomiting. *E. coli* is the most common cause found in developing countries. High-risk destinations include Latin America, Africa, the Middle East, and Asia. The risk is lower in some of the Caribbean islands.

Contaminated food or water—or both—is the cause. Cooked and raw foods can be implicated, most especially raw shellfish and raw fruits and vegetables. Where the food is prepared appears to be an important variable, with private homes, restaurants, and street vendors listed in order of increasing risk.

Rotaviruses and Norwalk virus are viral enteric pathogens that have become well known in recent years as the cruise ship virus. In fact, there were twenty-three outbreaks on cruise ships in 2002. Some cruise ships have had consecutive outbreaks, so before you book a cruise, ask how many times it has happened. On the ships the disease is not necessarily spread via the food, but through faulty handling of the food, or bad dishwashing procedures. Noroviruses spread through casual contact, such as picking up a poker chip, and they can survive outside the body for days. These viruses tend to break out not only on cruise ships but also in campgrounds, military camps, and overcrowded institutions. As much as 36 percent of diarrheal illness of travelers is associated with rotavirus in the stool.

Drink only bottled water and beverages. Avoid ice cubes or any foods and beverages prepared or washed with the local water supply. For example, you might be tempted to bite into a juicy piece of fruit, but if it was only rinsed off under the tap, it could be a source of trouble for you—unless you peel it. One of the ironies of getting travelers' diarrhea, of course, is that you need to keep replacing fluids in your body so you don't become dehydrated. This puts more stress on you to find beverages that can be consumed without causing even more problems.

Most over-the-counter antidiarrheal drugs are not effective in preventing travelers' diarrhea, but Pepto-Bismol taken every day has been shown to work in about 60 percent of cases in several studies. Ask your doctor before you take this because there are side effects to consider. They include temporary blackening of the tongue and stools, occasional nausea, and constipation. Don't take this if you have an aspirin allergy, renal insufficiency, or gout, or if you are taking heart or cancer medications.

Wash your hands frequently and carry with you some packaged sanitized hand wipes. The bacteria that cause the problems are easily passed from hand to money to food.

Talk with your doctor about taking prophylactic antibiotics if you are going to a country with known problems.

Appendix: Resources

This is a directory of organizations that can help you with information. The first section includes organizations that provide information on the entire gastrointestinal system. Then there are groups that specialize in one area, such as liver or celiac disease.

The Gastrointestinal System

National Institute of Diabetes and Digestive and Kidney Diseases
National Digestive Diseases Information Clearinghouse (a service of the National Institutes of Health)
2 Information Way
Bethesda, MD 20892-3570
www.niddk.nih.gov
The NIH also has a National Library of Medicine at www.nim.nih.gov/medlineplus.

American College of Gastroenterology
4900 B South 31st Street
Arlington, VA 22206
Phone: 703-820-7400
Fax: 703-931-4520
www.acponline.org

American Gastroenterological Association
7910 Woodmont Avenue, 7th Floor
Bethesda, MD 20814
Phone: 301-654-2055
Fax: 301-652-3890
www.gastro.org

The Centers for Disease Control and Prevention
1600 Clifton Road
Atlanta, GA 30333
Phone: 404-639-3534 or 800-311-3435
www.cdc.gov

American Society for Gastrointestinal Endoscopy
1520 Kensington Road, Suite 202
Oak Brook, IL 60523
Phone: 630-573-0600
Fax: 630-573-0691
www.asge.org
info@asgeoffice.org
The ASGE can help you locate a gastrointestinal endoscopist through their Web site. Click on "Find an Endoscopist." They also provide information on various endoscopic procedures.

American Medical Association
515 No. State Street
Chicago, IL 60610
Phone: 800-621-8335 (toll-free)
www.ama-assn.org
Click on "Find a Doctor."

CastleConnolly.com
"Find a Doctor" link. Physician profiles are selected after peer nomination, extensive research, and careful review and screening by their own physician-directed research team.

American Academy of Family Physicians
11400 Tomahawk Creek Parkway
Leawood, KS 66221
Phone: 913-906-6000 or 800-274-2237
www.familydoctor.org

The Stomach

The Helicobacter pylori Foundation
www.helico.com
help@helico.com

The Small Intestine (Celiac Disease)

The Celiac Disease Foundation
13251 Ventura Boulevard
Studio City, CA 91604
Phone: 818-990-2354
Fax: 818-990-2379
www.celiac.org
cdf@celiac.org

The Celiac Sprue Association
P. O. Box 31700
Omaha, NE 68131
Phone: 877-CSA-4CSA
  (toll-free)
Fax: 402-558-1347
www.csaceliacs.org
celiacs@csaceliac.org

*The Celiac Disease and
  Gluten-Free Diet Support
  Page*
www.celiac.com

The Gluten-Free Pantry
P. O. Box 840
Glastonbury, CT 06033
Phone: 800-291-8386
  (toll-free)
Fax: 860-633-6853
www.glutenfree.com
pantry@glutenfree.com

*Gluten Intolerance Group of
  North America*
15110 10th Avenue SW
Seattle, WA 98166
Phone: 206-246-6652
Fax: 206-246-6531
www.gluten.net
info@gluten.net

*American Dietetic
  Association*
120 So. Riverside Plaza
Chicago, IL 60606-6995
Phone: 800-877-1600
  (toll-free)
www.eatright.org
hotline@eatright.org
Other sources: In the section on celiac disease in
  chapter 6 you will find
  several other sources on
  gluten-free living.

The Pancreas
*National Pancreas
  Foundation*
P.O. Box 15333
Boston, MA 02215
Phone: 866-726-2737 (toll-
  free)
Fax: 617-247-8746
www.pancreasfoundation.org

The Liver
American Liver Foundation
75 Maiden Lane
New York, NY 10038
Phone: 800-465-4837 (Go
  Liver) (toll-free)
Fax: 212-483-8179
www.liverfoundation.org
info@liverfoundation.org

*American Hemochromatosis
  Society*
4044 W. Lake Mary Blvd.
Lake Mary, FL 32746
Phone: 888-655-IRON
  (4766)
Fax: 407-333-1284
www.americanhs.org

*The Hemochromatosis
  Foundation*
P. O. Box 8569
Albany, NY 12208-0569
Phone: 518-489-0972
Fax: 518-489-0227
www.hemochromatosis.org

*National Organization of
  Rare Disorders, Inc.*
55 Kenosia Avenue
Danbury, CT 06813-1968
Phone: 800-999-6673
  (voice mail only)
Fax: 203-798-2291
www.rarediseases.org

*Wilson's Disease
  Association*
1802 Brookside Drive
Wooster, OH 44691
Phone: 800-399-0266 (toll-
  free)
Fax: 509-757-6418
www.wilsonsdisease.org
info@wilsonsdisease.org

The Colon
*The Crohn's and Colitis
  Foundation of America*
386 Park Avenue South
New York, NY 10016
Phone: 800-932-2423
  (toll-free)
www.ccfa.org
info@ccfa.org

*The American Society of
  Colon and Rectal
  Surgeons*
85 W. Algonquin Road
Arlington Heights, IL
  60005
Phone: 847-290-9184
Fax: 847-290-9203
www.fascrs.org
ascrs@fascrs.org

*International Foundation
  for Functional Gastro-
  intestinal Disorders*
P. O. Box 17864
Milwaukee, WI 53217
Phone: 414-964-1799
  or 888-964-2001
www.ifgd.org
iffgd@iffgd.org

Index

About the Authors

Paul Miskovitz, M.D., is Clinical Professor of Medicine at Weill Medical College of Cornell University and an attending physician at New York–Presbyterian Hospital. Dr. Miskovitz practices gastroenterology in New York City.

Marian Betancourt is the author of several books, including *What to Do When Love Turns Violent,* and *Playing Like a Girl: Transforming Our Lives through Team Sports.* She is the coauthor of a dozen health books, including *The Prostate Cancer Sourcebook.* Ms. Betancourt lives in New York City.